HOW TO
feel great
ALL THE TIME

HOW TO
feel great
ALL THE TIME

A LIFELONG PLAN *for* UNLIMITED
ENERGY *and* RADIANT GOOD HEALTH

VALERIE SAXION

LION'S
HEAD
PUBLISHING

HOW TO FEEL GREAT ALL THE TIME

ISBN: 1-891668-17-X

Published by Lion's Head Publishing, 3 Coray Court,
Little Rock, AR 72223.

Literary development and cover/interior design
by Koechel Peterson & Associates, Minneapolis, Minnesota.

Manufactured in the United States of America.

DEDICATION

Jim,
my loving husband and father
of our seven children. You are truly
the sunshine of my life.
Thanks for how you have
encouraged me in my studies
in nutrition, but most importantly
for how you have sharpened
and inspired me in the Lord
and in His Word.

CONTENTS

Introduction   *xiii*

STEP ONE

WHEN IGNORANCE IS NOT BLISS

1 *A Guide to Understanding How Your Body Works*   3

2 *Junk Food*   19

3 *Body Oxygen*   29

4 *Exercise and Water*   43

STEP TWO

CLEANSE YOUR SYSTEM OF THE BAD STUFF

5 *Candida Albicans*   61

6 *Detoxification*   77

7 *Fasting*   93

STEP THREE

RESTORE YOUR SYSTEM TO GOD'S PLAN

8 *Reducing Your Temple Through Weight Loss*   109

9 *The One Perfect Diet—The Levitical Plan*   125

10 *Foods That Supercharge Your Mind and Body*   141

STEP FOUR

FINE-TUNE FOR YOUR SPECIFIC NEEDS

11 *Nature's Prescriptions for Feeling Great*   157

12 *Questions & Answers*   173

APPENDIX A: *America's Leading Complementary Alternative Medical Doctors*   191

APPENDIX B: *Silver Creek Laboratories Products*   243

ABOUT THE AUTHOR

DR. VALERIE SAXION IS ONE OF AMERICA'S MOST ARTICULATE CHAMPIONS OF NUTRITION AND SPIRITUAL HEALING. A twenty-year veteran of health science with a primary focus in Naturopathy, Valerie has a delightful communication style and charming demeanor that will open your heart, clear your mind, and uplift you to discover abundant natural health God's way. Her pearls of wisdom and life-saving advice are critical for success and survival in today's toxic world.

Dr. Saxion has avidly investigated and frequently advocated properly used oxygen, which she teaches, "has diminished in our atmosphere nearly 50 percent since creation." "It has a powerful capacity to prompt life and natural healing," she says, pointing to the longevity of Old Testament characters. And goes on to say, "This is really what the anti-aging baby boomers are looking for."

As the co-founder of Valerie Saxion's Silver Creek Labs, a manufacturer and distributor of nutritional supplements and health products with a spotlight on oxygenation, Dr. Saxion has seen firsthand the power of God's remedies as the sick are healed and the lame walk. "It's what I love most about what God has called me to do," she says.

Married to Jim Saxion for twenty-plus years, they are the parents of seven healthy children, ages 6 to 20.

After attending one of Dr. Saxion's lectures, you may have cried, you may have laughed, you may get insight, but one thing is sure: You will leave empowered with the tools to live and love in a healthy body!

Dr. Saxion has been interviewed on numerous radio talk shows as well as television appearances nationwide and in Canada. Hosts love to open the line for callers to phone in their health concerns while Dr. Saxion gives on-the-air advice and instruction.

She has also lectured at scores of health events nationwide and in Canada. She has advised international government leaders, professional athletes, television personalities, and the lady next door. "All with the same great results," she says, "if they will only follow the recommendations."

Dr. Saxion is currently a monthly columnist for BeautyWalk.com, hosted by Peter Lamas, famous makeup artist and hair designer for the rich and famous.

She is also a guest on the weekly Trinity Broadcasting Network program *Doctor to Doctor* that airs worldwide on TBN, Sky Angel, and the Health & Healing network.

To schedule Dr. Saxion for a lecture or interview, please contact Joy at 1-800-493-1146, or fax 817-236-5411, or email at valeriesaxon@cs.com.

Perhaps you are unfamiliar with the meaning of a naturopath, or N.D., such as Valerie Saxion. Michael Murray, who is probably the most well-known naturopath in the field, defines it in these terms:

"At the forefront of the natural medicine movement is Naturopathy, a method of healing that employs various natural means to empower an individual to achieve health. In addition to providing recommendations on life-style, diet, and exercise, naturopathic physicians may elect to utilize a variety of natural healing techniques, including clinical nutrition, herbal medicine, homeopathy, Oriental medicine and acupuncture, hydrotherapy, physical medicine, including massage and therapeutic manipulation and counseling.

"The modern naturopathic physician provides all phases of primary health care. He or she is trained to be the doctor first seen by the patient for general (non-emergency) health care. Some naturopathic physicians choose to emphasize a particular healing technique, while others are more eclectic and utilize a number of techniques. Some naturopaths elect to specialize in particular medical fields, such as pediatrics, natural childbirth, and physical medicine.

"Although the terms naturopathy and naturopathic medicine were not used until the late nineteenth century, their roots go back thousands of years. Drawing from the healing wisdom of many cultures, including India (Ayurvedic),

China (Taoist), and Greece (Hippocratic), naturopathic medicine is a system of medicine founded on the four time-tested medical principles—Naturopath, N.D.; Medical Doctor, M.D.; Osteopath, D.O.; and Chiropractor, D.C."

Dr. Saxion is a practicing Christian and does not adhere to occult practices or Eastern religions.

INTRODUCTION

We live on one-fourth of what we eat. Doctors live on the other three-fourths of what we eat.

INSCRIBED ON AN EGYPTIAN PYRAMID

WHEREVER I GO TO GIVE MY SEMINARS, WHENEVER I'M ON TELEVISION, AND WHENEVER I OPEN MY E-MAIL, THE CONSTANT COMPLAINT I GET IS THIS: "It's been a long time since I really felt good. I'm tired all the time. I'm exhausted and rundown. How can I start to feel good again?" My response is, "Why don't you feel *great all the time*? Why are you willing to settle for feeling less than 100 percent?"

My career and travels put me in contact with a great number of people, and I am amazed at how few people can tell me they are living in great health. When people discover that I am a naturopathic doctor, they typically launch into long lists of complaints about high blood pressure, high cholesterol, constant fatigue, headaches, a wide range of aches and pains, as well as fully developed diseases. Many spell out personal symptoms of diverse emotional problems, some of which have resulted in anger and frustration or feelings of hopelessness and depression.

They question me as though I have a magic vitamin

buried in my purse that will suddenly transport them to the land of radiant health. Perhaps I know of a wonder-working mineral or hormone that will make them all better? Or maybe I can tell them one thing they can do different to turn it all around?

Let me assure you that when I talk about feeling great all the time, there are no magic vitamins or minerals or hormones that do the trick. If you are experiencing a decline in health or a specific health problem, it usually has come on gradually and perhaps has been nearly undetectable. What is happening is that your body is sending you a signal that your body cells are in dis-ease. You have stepped out of homeostasis, "the state of being in health." Those body cells are not receiving the nutrients they need to sustain or propagate healthy cells, tissues, and organs. Dis-ease is associated generally with the absence or lack of some substance from our system, and/or a buildup of toxins in the bowels that needs to be eliminated.

Our typical response to the onset of a symptom or disease is to run to our medical doctor to get fixed, but doctors' prescriptions are seldom the "silver bullet" that answers the real problem. Too often we have been doing and are doing things to our bodies that cause the problems, and if these are left unresolved, our problems will persist or get worse. Years of abuse bring us to these points, and a quick and easy fix won't mend what's broken. It usually takes a complete program to provide your body with all the nutrients, minerals, exercise, and other sources it needs in sufficient and balanced quantities.

My intent is to not in any way discredit our extraordinary medical establishment within the United States. Nowhere in the world will you find a finer system of diagnosing disease. But even a casual observer will note that our national health system is severely lacking in the fields of nutrition and preventive medicine. Most of its focus has been and continues to be on dealing with symptoms of disease rather than stopping diseases from invading our bodies in the first place.

One does not have to be a doctor to see the problem. It usually can be seen by simply looking in a mirror. Most of us hope we can defy the laws of nature when it comes to our high-fat diets. On top of that, relatively few of us exercise, and millions of Americans abuse tobacco and alcohol despite prolific warnings. "Do not be deceived," the apostle Paul wrote two thousand ago, "God cannot be mocked. A man reaps what he sows" (Galatians 6:7). We're simply reaping the harvest we sowed by failing to treat our bodies with the respect they are due.

Correspondingly, the high rate of degenerative diseases in this country—such as heart attacks, cancers, strokes, cirrhosis of the liver, and emphysema—bears witness to the failure of medical prevention. As a society we have been incredibly slow to recognize the importance of weight loss, exercise, a healthy diet, as well as the value of vitamins, minerals, and herbal supplements. Until we actually put them to work in our lives and homes, we will never get close to feeling good all the time, let alone feeling great.

A staggering 70 percent of all deaths in this country are due to degenerative diseases. The Center for Disease Control has stated that 54 percent of heart disease, 50 percent of cerebrovascular disease (relating to or involving the blood vessels that supply the brain), 49 percent of atherosclerosis (a common arterial disease in which raised areas of degeneration and cholesterol deposits form on the inner surfaces of the arteries), and 37 percent of cancer are preventable through lifestyle changes. One needs to look no further than to poor nutrition as the leading preventable contributor to premature death in the United States.

You are mistaken if you think that you are in good health today because you are free from disease. If you are trying to get by with an unbalanced diet, your body may be able to cope for a lack of a specific nutritional substance for a while, but you can only cheat for so long and not pay a price. Eventually your system will not be able to rid itself of disease, and a health problem will surface. You may be fortunate enough to experience the early symptoms and seek effective treatment, but some people are not so fortunate. We cannot escape the fact that if we fail to supply our bodies with what they require to maintain the health of our cells, we will reap disease.

Besides the harm we may be doing to our bodies through poor diet habits and lack of exercise, there are other factors constantly warring against us—not all of which we can control. The effects of breathing in smog and cigarette smoke, exposing our bodies to increasing levels of UV rays, and contact with chemical products as well as their fumes have shown to cause damage to the cells of our bodies. We are surrounded by pesticides, asbestos, formaldehyde (in particle board, plywood, paints, and plastics), vinyl chloride, radioactivity, and X-rays—all of which are dangerous.

Add to that the preservatives and chemical additives to food, agricultural pesticides and hormone-enhancing drugs, chemical sprays, food processing, cured and processed meats, even our deodorants and shampoos, and the tremendous amounts of sugar added to our food. Government statistics state that the average American consumes a whopping 120 pounds of sugar each year, which is about 1/3 pound per day. Then there are the millions of daily stresses upon our lives that take their toll on our energies and health—emotional traumas of all sorts, physical injuries, crash diets and excessive exercising (to try to compensate for our lack of balance), allergies, antibiotics (that kill both bad and good bacteria in the body), and the fluctuations between hot and cold surroundings. All these negatively affect us over time, and one might think it a wonder that anyone is healthy.

There is good news, though, despite the bleak picture I've painted. Even if you have eaten badly since the day you were born and are suffering some bad effects in your body, God is a God of restoration. He has made your body in such a wonderful way that it is ceaselessly trying to make and keep you well. There is hope for every situation . . . even yours. At any moment, 50 percent of your cells are alive, 25 percent are dying off, and 25 percent are dead—this is a phenomenal process of regeneration. Your body is making billions of new cells right now. It is so efficient that if you are eating right, your liver regenerates itself every 7 days. It is actually possible to clean your body quickly and build health back into all your organs.

As long as those new body cells are being manufactured, you can make a difference in your health. These cells reach into your bloodstream to obtain more than 50 chemicals: amino acids (the building blocks of protein), fatty acids, minerals, trace elements, vitamins, and enzymes. These chemicals come from the food you eat, the water you drink, and the air you breathe—all of which you can do something about.

This book will teach you the basic things you can do to give your body the opportunity to start feeling great. Perhaps it starts with something as simple as eliminating junk food and drinking more water. It need not be complicated or expensive, and it doesn't necessitate becoming a vegetarian. It is totally doable, and you can start right where you are today.

Your attitude determines how great you can feel. If you want unbounded energy and an abundance of health in your everyday life, it begins with simple choices only you have the power to make.

I challenge you to take charge of your health and declare: *Today, I will start to get out of my box and find out how to get healthy. I will not allow any more excuses to keep me trapped in an unhealthy body or lifestyle. This is my life and my body, and I want it to be pleasing to God in every way.*

WHEN IGNORANCE IS NOT BLISS

*"My people
are destroyed
from lack of
knowledge"*

HOSEA 4:6

A GUIDE TO UNDERSTANDING HOW YOUR BODY WORKS

> *For you created my inmost being; you knit me together in my mother's womb. I praise you because I am fearfully and wonderfully made; your works are wonderful, I know that full well.*
>
> PSALM 139:14-15

LOUIS PASTEUR ONCE SAID, "THE MORE I STUDY NATURE, THE MORE I AM AMAZED AT THE CREATOR." I have been struck by the same reality when I study the human body in all its intricacies and complexities, particularly the immune system. God created us with an amazing healing system that is capable of handling almost any infection or disease. Our immune system provides for the efficient restoration of health as long as it is supported by the proper amounts of nutrition it requires.

Once upon a time in schools far away, we were taught about how our physical bodies work as well as the importance of nutrition and exercise. Perhaps we were too young to grasp the importance of the message delivered by our health teachers and the potential dire consequences of not putting that knowledge of the food pyramid into practice. Or perhaps our mother's deep fat fried chicken, French fries, soft drink, and sweet caramel rolls erased it from our minds. Yet we learned enough so that we tell ourselves over and over again that we know better than to keep abusing our bodies in the ways that we do.

So let's revisit what we heard long ago. If you hope to maintain your health, the quality of your nutrition directly influences your biochemistry as well as your immune system. Health and nutrition go hand in hand. Whether it involves bacteria, viruses, or fungi, there are many harmful microorganisms that constantly work to suppress the immune system. This can leave you more vulnerable to getting sick and make you susceptible to many diseases. The prevalence of the flu and colds and mononucleosis and bronchitis and yeast infections represent but a fraction of the problem we face today. It is said that by eating just 3 tablespoons of sugar you compromise your immune system up to 6 hours.

Where does the breakdown start? Again, it doesn't require a doctor to figure it out. Statistics from the United States Department of Agriculture show that as many as one out of every two Americans is not getting the minimum RDAs (Recommended Dietary Allowances) from their current diet. Keep in mind that these guidelines were established as a minimal level, not for maximizing your health! Meanwhile, other statistics show that fat consumption has increased by 30 percent and sugar consumption by 50 percent in the past several decades. It's a formula ripe for disease.

My hope is that the following snapshots of how your body works will help you come to grips with how you are living your life and what you are providing or depriving your body with regard to its healing and restoration. I would love it if the old proverb "an ounce of prevention is worth a pound of cure" becomes emblazoned on your mind.

THE AMAZING HEART

The human heart is one of the most amazing organs that God designed. It is the wondrous pump that powers the human body. It is a large, hollow, muscular organ divided into two pumps that lie side by side. Veins transport blood from throughout the body to the right-sided pump. That pump sends the blood to the lungs, where it picks up oxygen. The oxygenated blood then flows to the left side of the heart, which pumps it through arteries to the rest of the body. Valves control the flow of blood through the heart.

Our heart beats an average 70 times per minute, 100,000 times a day, 36.5 million times a year, and 2.5 billion times in a 68-year lifetime. Approximately 2.5 ounces of blood are pumped through the heart with every heartbeat—which means 1,080 gallons every day and 27 million gallons in an average lifetime. Is it any wonder that the condition of the heart is vital to feeling great all the time?

Despite unprecedented advancements in heart research and treatment, 1.5 million Americans will suffer a heart attack this year. Of that number, 300,000 will die before they reach a hospital or receive medical attention. Many of these heart attacks began with "The Silent Killer," or hypertension—abnormally high blood pressure accompanied by arterial disease. To understand it, you need a quick lesson about the heart.

When we have our blood pressure checked, it is measuring the actual force exerted by the blood against the walls of our blood vessels. It is our blood pressure that forces oxygen or plasma—which carries vitamins, minerals, glucose, amino acids, and fatty acids—into the body tissues through porous, microscopic capillary walls. Each person's blood pressure reflects the amount of blood in the body, the strength and rate of the heart's contractions, and the elasticity of the arteries.

Maintaining a normal blood pressure is crucial to the nutrition of the cells and tissues, providing a constant bathing in fresh, nutrient-laden RBCs (red blood cells) as well as removing the breakdown products from worn-out cells. The heart helps regulate blood pressure by producing a hormone that aids the kidneys in eliminating salt from the body. Excess salt may contribute to high blood pressure or hypertension. Hypertension can injure the heart, brain, and kidneys. Over many years, it can damage arteries and lead to heart disease.

When larger amounts of oxygen and nutrients are needed, the contraction of tiny muscles in the arterial walls causes the pressure to increase and supplies to be pushed more quickly to the cells. On the other hand, if few nutrients are required, these muscles relax, the pressure decreases, and food is conserved.

The most common heart disease affects the arteries that supply the heart muscle itself with blood. Disorders of those arteries usually develop over a person's lifetime. Deposits of fatty material block the arteries and so reduce the blood supply to the heart. If the heart muscle receives insufficient blood, it may work poorly or even die. Damage to the heart muscle resulting from a shortage of blood is called a heart attack. A mild heart attack may force a person to lead a less active life. A severe attack may make the heart unable to supply the body with enough blood even at rest and cause a person's death.

THE LUNGS

The right and left lungs are the chief breathing organs of the body. Their main job is to exchange gases. A lung has a spongy texture and may be thought of as an elastic bag filled with millions of tiny air chambers or sacs. Each sac contains about 20 tiny air spaces called alveoli. The walls of each alveolus contain networks of extremely small blood vessels called pulmonary capillaries. The alveolar walls are so thin that oxygen and carbon dioxide move through them easily. It is here that gas exchange takes place. As blood flows through the lungs, it picks up oxygen from the air and releases carbon dioxide. The body needs oxygen to burn food for energy, and it produces carbon dioxide as a waste product.

Because the lungs must inhale the air from the environment, they are exposed to bacteria, viruses, dust, and a variety of pollutants. The lungs have an efficient system via mucus and special cells called alveolar macrophages to eliminate these invaders, but the system can be overwhelmed. Cigarette smoke, air pollution, asbestos, silica, and coal dust are but a few contributors. Emphysema, asthma, and chronic bronchitis cause the airways to become partly blocked or narrower, making it more difficult for air to move through them. Infectious lung diseases, such as tuberculosis and pneumonia, are caused by bacteria, viruses, or other organisms.

With gas exchange occurring at such an extraordinarily vulnerable spot, it is easy to understand how crucial the health of the lungs and the blood system is to the overall health of our bodies.

THE LIVER AND KIDNEYS

Every cell in our body has the ability to take in harmful chemicals and detoxify them (to remove the poison or transform the toxin into something harmless). But the major organ of detoxification within the body is the liver. It is the largest gland in the human body and one of the most complex of all human organs. The liver serves as the body's main chemical factory and is one of its major storehouses of food.

The liver performs many essential functions. One of its most important tasks is to help the body digest food. It produces and secretes bile into the small intestine, where it aids in the digestion of fats. It also takes part in many metabolic functions, such as the conversion of sugars into glycogen, which it releases into the blood when the body needs it. It is your primary storage and distribution center for food. The liver plays an essential role in the storage of vitamins A, D, E, and K, and those of the B-complex group, as well as minerals and iron, and distributes 90 percent of all your nutrients to their destinations. In addition, the liver filters poisons and waste products from the blood.

Located in the upper right part of the abdominal cavity, your liver receives about three pints of blood for cleansing every minute of the day. Most of the food that we eat is taken in the blood straight from the intestine to the liver for detoxification, and only then is released for circulation to the rest of the body. Both the quality of the nutrition received as well as the condition of the liver to cleanse the blood are critical for optimal health.

The liver removes dangerous foreign particles from your system—whether it is dead or abnormal cells, yeasts, bacteria, viruses, parasites, incompletely digested or abnormal proteins, or artificial chemicals. Hormones are also taken out of circulation once they have completed their functions, and the dangerous ammonia that is formed when aged proteins are broken down is taken out by our liver, which converts it to urea and sends it off to the kidneys to be discharged in urine.

As might be expected, the liver is often the first organ to suffer when our detoxification systems become overwhelmed. For example, when a person is constipated, the liver has to work twice as hard to maintain the same level. Not only can it get to the place where it can no longer perform its detoxification tasks, but its numerous functions also suffer, causing many different symptoms.

The kidneys are a pair of organs in the abdomen that perform many vital functions, of which the most important is the production of urine. They filter waste liquid resulting from metabolism of the blood and remove a number of toxins, including urea, which the liver has changed so that they dissolve in water. If the kidneys fail to function, poisons build up in the body and eventually cause death. Our kidneys work best when we drink plenty of good clean water.

THE BRAIN

Weighing in at less than three pounds, the brain is the control center of our body's central nervous system, connected to the spinal cord and enclosed in the cranium. It consists of a compact network of more than ten billion nerve cells, nerve tissue, and nerve-supporting and nourishing tissue (neuroglia). The brain is the center of thought and emotions and regulates bodily activities. It is one of the busiest, most metabolically active organs in the body and is made up of approximately 65 percent fat.

Despite its size, the brain is involved in 15 percent of the body's total blood flow, 25 percent of its oxygen utilization, and at least 70 percent of its glucose (sugar) consumption. Unlike other organs, the brain is not capable of storing its own supply of energy. It depends, rather, on a constant flow of blood to keep it supplied with the nutrients it needs. While other organs in the body can metabolize fat and protein for energy, the brain must depend primarily on glucose from the blood for energy. Thus the reason why you get brain fog when you don't eat or don't eat properly.

Deprived of the proper nutrients in the bloodstream, proteins used by nerve cells in the brain cannot be manufactured, which can lead to the impairment of mental functions such as memory as well as a person's mood. It must have a continual supply of glucose, oxygen, and other essential nutrients. Also, unlike other tissues in the body that can heal after an injury, brain cells are incapable of regenerating themselves. This makes the brain especially vulnerable to illness and injury.

The brain can go without oxygen for only three to five minutes before serious damage results. A stroke results from the stoppage of the blood flow to the brain. There is either a sudden blockage or a rupture of a blood vessel to the brain, which results in the possible loss of consciousness, partial loss of movement, or loss of speech. It is thus a blood vessel disease—the cerebral (brain) equivalent of a heart attack. Most strokes result from damage to the blood vessels caused by high blood pressure or hardening of the arteries.

Strokes are the third most frequent cause of death in the United States among adults and the most common cause of neurological disability. Strokes and other cerebrovascular disorders affect about 500,000 Americans every year, with more than two-thirds of these patients being 65 or older. Because more aggressive therapies for high blood pressure and heart disease have been developed and used in the last 30 years, stroke deaths have dropped. Still, the mortality rate for those afflicted is high. An estimated one in four stroke patients dies within a month of their brain injury.

THE EYE

The eye is the organ of sight. It is our most important organ for finding out about the world around us. We use our eyes for almost everything we do. But the eye itself does not actually see objects. Instead, it sees the light they reflect or give off. Light rays enter the eye through transparent tissues. The eye changes the rays into electrical signals. The signals are then sent by the optic nerve to the brain, which interprets them as visual images.

Every waking second the light-sensitive rod and cone cells in the retina of the eye send about a billion pieces of fresh information to the brain for interpretation. The eye can sense about ten million gradations of light and seven million gradations of color. We see in such detail because the eye is almost an extension of our brain.

The health of the eye is largely dependent on a variety of nutrients, the foremost of which is oxygen. When the normal functions that deliver nutrition and oxygen to the eye begin to fail, many disorders follow—cataracts, glaucoma, macular degeneration. Antioxidants seem to offer the greatest protection against age-related degeneration of the eyes.

THE SKIN

Your skin is the largest organ of the human body. It protects the body in a wide variety of ways. For example, the skin is almost completely waterproof and so prevents the escape of the fluids that bathe the body's tissues. It also prevents bacteria and chemicals from entering most parts of the body. The skin also protects underlying tissues from harmful rays of the sun. In addition, the skin helps keep the internal temperature of the body within normal levels. Glands in the skin release sweat when a person becomes overheated. It breathes and releases toxins if necessary through perspiration.

When we think of our skin, we probably think of safeguarding ourselves from burns, damage from ultraviolet light, psoriasis, and acne. But what most people don't realize is that whatever you put on your skin is absorbed into your bloodstream. So read the labels and be aware of the chemicals that make contact with your skin. If there are harmful chemicals in our household cleaners, makeups, creams, deodorants, etc., they *will* find their way into our blood.

THE ADRENAL GLANDS

The two adrenal glands are endocrine glands perched atop each of our kidneys. The hormones they produce are essential for life. These hormones regulate the use of digested foods and help the body adapt to stress, regulate the excretion of sodium and potassium by the kidneys, and produce small amounts of sex hormones.

The inner part of each gland secretes epinephrine (adrenalin), and the outer part secretes norepinephrine (noradrenalin) into the blood. These hormones help the body adjust to sudden stress and prepare us for "fight or flight." For example, they increase the speed and strength of the heartbeat and raise the blood pressure.

Stresses tend to overstimulate or whip the adrenal glands to produce cortisone. When this happens, vital calcium is pulled from the body's bones, sugar from the liver, and protein from the muscles. Over time, stress exhausts the adrenals to the point where no "whip" is big enough to get them going again in an adequate way.

BONES

Nearly half of the women between the ages of 45 and 75 show signs of some degree of osteoporosis, which is a loss of bone tissue, and over a third suffer from serious bone deterioration. Osteoporosis can result from various hormonal diseases, local injury or inflammation, and lack of physical activity, as well as the natural loss of bone that occurs as a person grows older. The most common form of osteoporosis affects women who are past menopause.

To prevent osteoporosis, physicians recommend a life-long combination of regular exercise and a diet high in calcium. It was reported that the current National Health Care Cost in this country could be reduced by $16 billion dollars if women would take a supplement of just 1,000 milligrams of calcium a day. More than one million hip fractures occur in women over the age of only 45, and many older patients die of complications. One's bone density today determines their skeletal strength tomorrow.

PROTEIN

Protein is one of the three main classes of nutrients that provide energy to the body (the others are carbohydrates and fats), and I highlight them because of their importance in regard to nutrition. Proteins exist in every cell and are essential to life. We must obtain most of them from the foods we eat.

Proteins are large, complex molecules made up of small

units called amino acids. The amino acids are linked together into long chains called polypeptides. Twenty amino acids are assembled into the thousands of different proteins required by the human body. To assemble the proteins it needs, the body must have a sufficient supply of all these amino acids. Some amino acids, called essential amino acids, cannot be produced by the body and must be supplied by various foods. Humans require nine essential amino acids. The remaining acids, called nonessential amino acids, can be manufactured by the body itself.

When protein is eaten, your digestive processes break it down into amino acids, which pass into the blood and are carried throughout the body. Your cells can then select the amino acids they need for the construction of tissue repair and new body tissue (especially bone cartilage and muscle), antibodies, hormones, enzymes, and worn-out and dead blood cells. Every cell needs protein to maintain its life. The importance of this is seen in these examples:

■ Most white blood cells are replaced every 10 days.
■ The cells in the line of the gastrointestinal tract and blood platelets are replaced every 4 days.
■ Skin cells are replaced every 24 days.
■ More than 98 percent of the molecules in the body are completely replaced every year.

Your muscles, hair, nails, skin, and eyes are made of protein. So are the cells that make up the liver, kidneys, heart, lungs, nerves, brain, and your sex glands. The body's most active protein users are the hormones secreted from the various glands—thyroxin from the thyroid, insulin from the pancreas, and a variety of hormones from the pituitary—as well as the soft tissues, hardworking major organs, and muscles. They all require the richest stores of protein.

The complete proteins that contain the essential amino acids come from meat, poultry, fish, eggs, milk—all dairy products. Cereal grains, nuts, legumes (peas and beans), and vegetables contain some but not all of the essential amino acids.

Insufficient protein in the diet may cause a lack of energy, stunted growth, and lowered resistance to disease. If the body does not receive enough proteins from the food eaten, it uses proteins from the cells of the liver and muscle tissues. Continued use of such proteins by the body can permanently damage those tissues. You don't want that to happen.

SO WHAT'S THE POINT?

The point is simple. Your body is wonderfully made and totally interconnected. If you are careful to supply it with all that it absolutely requires for health, whether by nutrients or exercise, radiant health will reign over every aspect of your body. You will begin to feel great physically and emotionally! You will have unlimited energy to do all the things you want and be the person you want to be.

But if you fall short, if you deprive your body of those essentials or abuse your body with what you know or don't know is harmful, you will suffer a breakdown in your health, and that specific symptom will negatively affect your whole person. It's inescapable! All of your energies will be burned in trying to cope with the disease, and it will significantly limit all you wish to do as well as the person you'd like to be.

The choice is yours.

JUNK FOOD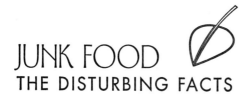
THE DISTURBING FACTS

Nature is doing her best each moment to make us well. She exists for no other end. Do not resist. With the least inclination to be well, we should not be sick.

HENRY DAVID
THOREAU

"JUNK FOOD" IS A GENERAL TERM THAT HAS COME TO ENCOMPASS FOODS THAT OFFER LITTLE IN TERMS OF PROTEIN, MINERALS, OR VITAMINS, AND LOTS OF CALORIES FROM SUGAR OR FAT. While there is no definitive list of junk foods, most authorities include foods that are high in salt, sugar, or fat calories, and low nutrient content. The big hitters on most people's lists include fried fast food, salted snack foods, carbonated beverages, candies, gum, and most sweet desserts. The term "empty calories" reflects the lack of nutrients found in junk food.

According to a recent study in the *American Journal of Clinical Nutrition*, one-third of the average American's diet is made up of junk foods. Because junk foods take the place of healthier foods, these same Americans are depending on the other two-thirds of their diet to get 100 percent of the recommended dietary intake of vitamins and nutrients. Studies show that the average American gets 27 percent of their total daily energy from junk foods and an additional 4 percent from alcoholic beverages. About one-third of Americans consume an average of 45 percent of energy from these foods. Researchers are certain that such patterns of eating may have long-term, even life-threatening, health consequences.

If you have any question about the nutritional value of a food, judge it by the list of ingredients and the Nutrition Facts label found on packages. That label will list the number of calories per serving, grams of fat, sodium, cholesterol, fiber, and sugar content. If sugar, fat, or salt show up as one of the first three ingredients, you can probably consider that food to be a nutritional risk.

KICKING THE HABIT

If you've made hundreds of resolutions, vowing to kick the junk-food habit, only to fail over and over again, you're not alone. In fact, many people have simply given up on making resolutions altogether.

Well, I've got good news. You can kick the junk-food habit, but you can't do it alone. You need "the God factor" at work in you in order to achieve a strong, healthy body. I've learned that truth over the years, and that's why I sought the Lord on this junk-food matter. I wanted to help those who were crying out to me, wanting to change their eating habits and become healthier—in control of their health instead of being controlled. And this is what the Lord gave me—a plan to kick that junk-food habit once and for all!

Read on to learn the steps that will set you free from junk food and empower you to walk in health and fulfill the desires of your heart!

TAKING DOMINION

I want to give you a revelation—nothing should have dominion over you! Did you know that? But if you are being driven by coffee, cigarettes, cakes, candy, or lust of any kind, that thing has a hold on you! The Bible says that God has given us spiritual authority over anything that tries to control us! So if we have that authority, we need to act on it. Here's how you do it.

1. **Realize there's a problem!** The first step to utilizing your spiritual authority over food or whatever has a hold on you is admitting you have a problem.

2. **Ask for the Holy Spirit's help!** Ask the Holy Spirit to reveal anything that is not pleasing to Him. If you really want to be free, listen when He answers. You may be surprised at what He reveals to you.

3. **Repent!** Ask the Lord to forgive you for allowing food to have such a strong hold on your life, and thank Him for showing you this area of your life that needs work. Don't beat yourself up over it. Just repent and receive God's forgiveness and love.

4. **Obtain grace!** Go boldly before the throne of God to obtain grace—grace that will help you in times of need (Hebrews 4:16). He has enough grace for every situation, so don't sweat it!

5. **Ask for wisdom!** God knows you better than you know yourself, and He knows what it will take to get you out of bondage. So ask Him for wisdom concerning your particular food struggle. He wants you free, and "if the Son sets you free, you will be free indeed" (John 8:36).

DEALING WITH THE ROOT

Now it's time to deal with the root of your addictions! Many times the root is not what you think it is. Certainly, there is a spirit of gluttony in the earth today, but I believe a lot of Christians are battling a physical problem—not just a spiritual one.

For instance, some people crave sweets and sugary foods because they have a *Candida Albicans* problem, not a lack of willpower or a spirit of gluttony. You may fall into this category and not even be aware of it. I have dedicated an entire chapter to this problem because I feel it is so universally prevalent. I will only briefly touch on it here.

Candida Albicans is a yeastlike fungus that can run rampant in a person eating the typical American diet of sugars, high carbohydrates, alcohol, etc., and who has been on even a couple rounds of antibiotics over the years. In the United States a large percentage of the 40 million prescriptions written each week are for antibiotics. When you take an antibiotic, you not only kill the bad bacteria, but you kill the good bacteria, the good intestinal flora that God put in your body. And flora is vital for a healthy immune system. So if you do not take a probiotic each time you have been on an antibiotic, you are setting yourself up for *Candida*.

How does this relate to junk foods? It means that if you have this yeastlike fungus in your system, it needs to be fed. And believe me, it will tell you what to eat! It may scream for sugar, pickled foods, breads, and even alcohol. Yes, I said alcohol! I believe that *Candida* can be a factor in what drives some people to drink.

Many years ago I heard about a study that said chil__ who craved sweets had a significantly higher chance of becoming addicted to alcohol as adults. On the surface, you might think compulsive behavior, right? But here's my take on it: I think there is a driving force. That force is *Candida*. It can start as a child and totally change the outcome of one's life if not dealt with.

Not understanding yeast and bacteria in the body can cause you to be looking in the wrong direction for your answers. Maybe your junk-food craving is *Candida*-driven. Some of the *Candida* symptoms are heartburn, indigestion, gas, itching, yeast infections, Jock itch, athlete's foot, post nasal drip, headaches, mucous in stools, dry mouth, bad breath, and the list goes on! If you suffer from those symptoms, consider going on a *Candida* cleanse for 30-60 days. In severe cases it may require 90-120 days. It certainly won't hurt you, and it might really help!

Remember, wisdom is the principal key! God's wisdom far exceeds what we can even think or imagine. So seek Him in everything, and ask Him to direct your path on your way to a strong, healthy body—a body that is free from bondage and able to serve Him without fatigue or pain.

EXERCISE, WATER, AND OXYGENATE YOUR WAY TO HEALTH

Exercise, water, and oxygen are so important to your overall health that you need to study my chapters dedicated specifically to these. Please read those to fill in the bigger picture of the value you'll gain by taking these seriously.

While most of us are not trying to achieve model-like figures or body-builder physiques, we should exercise for general health purposes. According to the American Heart Association, participating in regular aerobic (with oxygen) exercise decreases your risk of heart attacks and strokes. Exercise also relieves stress. And exercise increases your metabolism, energy level, immunity, and oxygen level, while helping you look and feel better. Especially important to the junk-food problem, exercise also decreases your appetite. So hit the treadmill, not the candy store. You will be amazed at how this will help to cut your cravings and give you more energy immediately.

Water, water, water! You can't get enough! Did you know that you are 65 percent water? On the whole, people are not replenishing the very element God put in them. We should be drinking at least half our body weight in ounces of steam-distilled water to pull out and strip the toxins that build up in the body. And here's another benefit of drinking water. It will help rid your body of those awful cravings. As the water flushes out your system, it cleanses the remainder of any junk food you've eaten. Did you know that the last food you ate will be the next food you crave? So if you are loading up with junk food, you will continue craving it if you do not get it flushed out of your system. It's a vicious cycle.

Increasing your oxygen levels will speed up your metabolism. And when you get that natural high from oxygen, you'll be less likely to crave artificial energy boosters such as caffeine, sugar, and carbohydrates. Not only will increased oxygen give you more energy, it will also promote a better mental attitude, make you more alert, and give your thought processes more definition. Then, you can think it through before grabbing a snack, soda, or coffee.

STEP BY STEP

Since you know your goal, I've got an assignment for you. Make a list of the junk foods, sugary drinks, caffeine-packed foods and drinks, and other toxic foods and beverages that you want to eliminate from your life.

Next, get a calendar and lay out a plan to delete one thing at a time from your current eating habits.

- Week One—switch from table salt to sea salt. And begin reading the ingredients on everything you buy. If you don't know what it is, don't eat it!
- Week Two—replace bleached flour with unbleached flour. And refuse to eat anything with artificial flavoring or coloring.
- Week Three—switch from black pepper to cayenne or paprika.
- Week Four—determine to drink at least 64 ounces (or one half your body weight in ounces) of steam-distilled water every day.
- Week Five—replace your coffee habit with herbal teas.
- Week Six—switch from donuts, cookies, and muffins to a healthy, flavorful protein bar (low in carbohydrates and high in protein).
- Week Seven—schedule your five fruits and veggies per

day, one week at a time. Plan to take in only fresh snacks.

- For one entire week refuse to go to a fast-food restaurant, and then just keep the resolve.
- Another week, determine to eat nothing fried.
- As soon as possible switch over and begin to plan your meals on a weekly basis from the One Perfect Levitical Diet in chapter 9. I know this will make a huge difference in how you feel.

This list is just the beginning. You write the rest of the story based on your personal needs and challenges because only you know where your food addictions lie. If you have a specific food that troubles you, find a delicious, healthy alternative!

Write your vision, and go for it one step at a time. It's a cinch by the inch, but a trial by the mile.

PRAYER AND FASTING

Fasting should have a place in our lives for spiritual and physical reasons. Pray about going on the fasting and detoxing program I have laid out in chapter 7 of this book. Isaiah 58 says that "by fasting, your health will spring forth speedily," and that certainly applies to getting out of the junk-food habit. Isaiah also says that fasting will loose the bands of wickedness, undo the heavy burdens, let the oppressed go free, and break every yoke. Being in bondage to food can control your life. Consider fasting as a weapon—a force to break the junk-food habit once and for all!

The benefits of fasting are similar to the benefits of

using the best gas in your car. You stop sputtering around and start firing on all cylinders. Fasting will pull out those harmful toxins that are driving you to crave and eat foods you know aren't good for you, and fasting will cleanse your system so you won't eat the foods you really don't want. And, it does it fast, speedily, as the Word says. I've seen absolute miracles in just four days. Maybe you will be my next testimonial.

PREPARATION BRINGS VICTORY

In this war against junk food or other addictions in your life, you must have a strategy for success. Preparation is a major key! So prepare in advance! Failure to plan is a plan to fail!

Always make sure you have healthy snacks available, such as fruits, raisins, yogurt, nuts, carrots, celery sticks, smoothies, etc. If you have something healthy on hand, it's easy! If not, when hunger strikes, you will be tempted to grab the closest, quickest thing you can get your hands on, which probably won't be good for you.

Fast-food restaurants and convenience stores have made millions of dollars based on this fact. They are on every street corner just waiting for your stomach to growl. They will take advantage of you if you are unprepared. So be ready in season and out, as the Word says (2 Timothy 4:2). Have something good on hand, or learn to do without, which isn't such a bad idea either.

If, for example, you know that your worst snacking time falls between 5 P.M. and 6 P.M., there's probably a reason for that. Maybe your blood sugar is low at that time of day, prompting you to eat uncontrollably as you prepare dinner for the rest of the family. So eat a piece of fruit on the way home from work—plan ahead!

YOU CAN DO IT!

Many blessings to you as you endeavor to kick the junk-food habit. It's all a part of restoring the beautiful temple that God gave you! No matter what shape your body is in right now, you can start today and begin seeing results. You can do it! I say that confidently because I've seen God work miracles in my life and many others using these same tips and informational guidelines.

God wants to help you attain a healthy and fit body—just ask Him. He will help you grow in self-control, patience, and the other fruit of the Spirit (Galatians 5:22-23) that you'll need to win this war. You can do it because you're not alone. You have the God of the universe on your side, and we're praying for your success, too!

As always, consult your physician before starting any new exercise or diet program. But start where you are! Educate yourself. You are your best physician!

BODY OXYGEN

> *The Lord God formed the man from the dust of the ground and breathed into his nostrils the breath of life, and the man became a living being.*
>
> GENESIS 2:7

SINCE THE CREATION OF THE WORLD, OXYGEN HAS BEEN AND CONTINUES TO BE THE VERY BREATH OF LIFE THAT KEEPS EVERY ONE OF US FUNCTIONING FOR OUR ALLOTTED SPACE OF TIME UPON THIS PLANET. Genesis 2:7 tells us that God made man out of the dust of the earth and then breathed into his nostrils "the breath of life," after which "man became a living being."

Taber's Cyclopedic Medical Dictionary states that oxygen is essential to the respiration of most forms of animal and plant life, and is the most important and abundant element, composing about 21 percent of the atmosphere's total volume. It is absorbed by plants in the form of water and carbon dioxide, which are converted into organic substances utilized for the food of man, and in turn is returned to the atmosphere by man in form of waste products of water and carbon dioxide, thus maintaining the balance of oxygen and carbon dioxide in the atmosphere.

Taber's also states that in conditions in which there is insufficient oxygen being carried by the blood to our body tissues, oxygen is to be used in cases of severe anemia, shock, circulatory collapse, pulmonary edema, pneumonia, and many others. A study of the wonders of oxygen quickly explains why this is.

THE WONDERS OF OXYGEN

Oxygen is your greatest and first source of energy. It is the fuel required for the proper operation of all your body systems. Only 10 percent of your energy comes from food and water; *90 percent of your energy comes from oxygen.* Oxygen gives your body the ability to rebuild itself. Oxygen detoxifies the blood and strengthens the immune system. Oxygen displaces or burns deadly free radicals, neutralizes environmental toxins, and destroys anaerobic (depleted of oxygen) bacteria, parasites, microbes, and viruses.

Oxygen greatly enhances the body's absorption of vitamins, minerals, amino acids, proteins, and other important nutrients. Oxygen enhances brain power and memory. Oxygen can beneficially affect your learning ability. The ability to think, feel, and act is all dependent on oxygen. It also calms the mind and stabilizes the nervous system. Oxygen heightens concentration and alertness. Without oxygen, brain cells die and deteriorate quickly. As you age, and oxygen deficiency increases, it takes longer to learn, and your retention span is decreased.

We can live for weeks without food. We can even live for a few days without water. But we can only live for minutes without oxygen. Oxygen strengthens the heart. Increased oxygen lowers the resting heart rate and strengthens the

contraction of the cardiac muscle. Corresp[...]
ally all heart attacks can be attributed to a fa[...]
oxygen to the heart muscle.

Oxygen treatments provide a safe, hi[...] [...]cctive
method for the recovery of oxygen to all body systems. The
effects are cumulative. The body begins to work more efficiently as it restores the oxygen balance closer to the higher
natural range it was originally designed to function with. It
helps reverse the physical and psychological effects of oxygen deprivation from poor health, air pollution, water pollution, food pollution, and aging.

Maintaining proper oxygen levels in the body is an
essential ingredient to health, vitality, physical stamina,
and endurance. You must have a means of replenishing
your oxygen level. Researchers, scientists, molecular biolo-
gists, nutritional specialists, and others have reported phenomenal health benefits from increased oxygen uptake.
World-class professional athletes, renowned fitness trainers,
coaches, and "average" citizens have also reported experiencing many of these benefits.

BENEFITS OF INCREASED OXYGEN

- Increases energy levels
- Increases stamina and endurance
- Enhances the absorption of vitamins, minerals, amino
  acids, proteins, and other important nutrients
- Rapid fatigue recovery
- Lowers resting heart rate
- Kills infectious bacteria, viruses, fungi, and parasites,

but does not harm the "good" microorganisms the body needs

- Relieves pain
- Improves circulation
- Improves sleep
- Strengthens the immune system
- Heightens concentration and alertness
- Increases fat metabolism resulting in a loss of body fat
- Calms the nervous system
- Improves memory
- Corrects chemical imbalances in the body
- Relieves headaches
- Accelerates healing time for injuries
- Lowers blood pressure
- Relieves stress and anxiety
- Allows the body to direct enough oxygen to its primary functions without having to draw on valuable reserves
- Helps reverse premature aging
- Relieves symptoms of PMS in women
- Helps displace damaging free radicals
- Helps neutralize harmful toxins in cells, tissues, and bloodstream

SO WHAT'S THE PROBLEM?

There are two very big problems concerning oxygen that may be killing you ever so slowly. According to Dr. Carl Baugh, noted archeologist, author, and creationist, in pre-flood conditions the oxygen saturation levels in the earth's atmosphere were 35 percent, and carbon dioxide was probably less than 1 percent. Today in "country living" you may get 21 percent oxygen. In "big city" pollution, we do good to get 17-18 percent oxygen with 25 percent carbon dioxide. The truth is that there is much *less oxygen in the air to breathe*, and what is there brings chemical pollutants and other harmful substances into our bodies.

The other major problem was highlighted in Paul Bragg's book *Super Power Breathing for Super Energy*. According to Bragg, most people are *starving the body of vital oxygen through their shallow breathing*. It is reported that people in Western cultures barely use one-fifth of the lung's capacity to increase the oxygen flow to their bodies. He attributes the headaches, muscular aches and pains, stiff joints, constipation, indigestion, aching backs and feet, poor eyesight, poor hearing, sore throats, and respiratory ailments such as emphysema, asthma, sinus infections, and bronchitis as directly linked to shallow breathing and leading to early graves.

Perhaps you think Bragg is too extreme? Listen to Dr. Philip C. Stavish's comments in an article in the *Journal of Longevity* that was titled "Oxygen Decrease Leading to Worldwide Increase in Disease." He concurs that we are slowly suffocating from a lack of oxygen and that oxygen deficiency causes everything from a feeling of uneasiness to full-blown disease. "Oxygen deficiency," he states, "results in a weakened immune system, which can lead to viral problems, damaged cell growth, toxic buildup in the blood, and premature aging—among other ailments."

According to Norman McVea, M.D., Ph.D., in *Wellness*

Lifestyle magazine, "More than anything else, good health and well-being is dependent on the maximum production, maintenance and flow of energy, which is produced by oxygen.... It contributes to proper metabolic function, better circulation, assimilation, digestion, and elimination. Oxidation is the key to life."

We take oxygen for granted, to the point we just aren't realizing that we need to increase our oxygen levels in *every way possible*. I was talking to a manager of a health food store one time and mentioned the products that our business has developed for oxygen supplementation. Her response was "I'm not into that oxygen stuff." Well, if you're not into it, you're probably dead or rapidly on your way.

THE REALLY BIG HEALTH PROBLEMS

First, there are *heart*-related problems due to the lack of oxygen in our systems. Virtually all heart attacks can be attributed to a failure to deliver oxygen to the heart muscle. Dr. Richard Lippman, renowned researcher, states that a lack of oxygen (hypoxia) is the prime cause of 1.5 million heart attacks each year. Research studies show that mild hypoxia increases the heart and respiratory rates; however, prolonged or severe hypoxia results in lung or heart failure.

Second, there are also *cancer*-related problems that arise. According to Dr. Carl Warburg, noted researcher and Nobel Prize winner in 1952, "Once the level of oxygen available in a cell drops below 60 percent of normal, the cell is forced to switch to an inferior method of energy production—fermentation. The cell can never be returned to the proper oxidation system and produces alcohol and lactic acid. If a parasite moves into the area and begins to feed on the alcohol, its waste products inhibit the suppressers of enzyme growth factor (EGF). The anaerobic cells are flooded with EGF and begin to replicate themselves wildly. This condition, we call cancer."

Dr. Warburg also pointed out that any substance that deprives a cell of oxygen is a carcinogen, if the cell is not killed outright. He stated that it is useless to search out new carcinogens, because the result of each one is the same—cellular deprivation of oxygen. He further stated that the incessant search for new carcinogens is counterproductive because it obscures the prime cause, a lack of oxygen, and prevents appropriate treatment. The National Cancer Institute endorsed Dr. Warburg's findings in 1952.

Dr. Harry Goldblatt published similar findings in the *Journal of Experimental Medicine* in 1953. His research confirmed that a lack of oxygen plays the major role in causing cells to become cancerous. "Disease is due to a deficiency in the oxidation process of the body, leading to an accumulation of toxins." Keep in mind these toxins are ordinarily burned in normal oxidation.

Dr. Wendell Hendricks of the Hendricks Research Foundation wrote, "Cancer is a condition within the body where the oxidation has become so depleted that the body cells have degenerated beyond control. The body is so overloaded with toxins that it sets up a tumor mass to harbor these poisons and remove them from general activity within the body."

Hulda Clark, noted speaker and author of *Cure for All Diseases,* states that there are two things that all cancer patients have in common: *They all lack oxygen,* and they are all loaded with parasites. That makes total sense when you see that one can lead to the other's existence. Cancer cells cannot live in an oxygen-rich environment.

A third major health concern regards *the burning of fat.* In Dr. Heinerman's *Encyclopedia of Nature's Vitamins & Minerals,* he states that oxygen is the key to burning stored fat. "If you want help in losing weight, stoke your biological furnace with more oxygen. The oxygen you take in is carried directly to cell mitochondria, where energy is created and preserved. Your body's internal combustion gets accelerated to the point that more stored fat is chemically burned off." This is because the highest grade fuel in the body is fat, or lipids. Additional oxygen that is brought into the body helps to burn that high-grade fuel.

All cells derive their energy from glucose. Healthy cells burn glucose in oxygen by oxidation, while unhealthy cells ferment glucose anaerobically, producing large amounts of lactic acid. Fermentation produces only one-sixth the energy of oxidation, so diseased cells are perpetually starving for energy and have huge appetites for sugar. This wasteful metabolism becomes self-sustaining and dominant unless the oxygen level is sharply increased.

Healthy cells that have sufficient oxygen and nutrients manufacture an enzyme coating around them that protects them from invasion. With the enzyme coating the cell is safe from invasion from viruses, and oxygen cannot harm it.

Oxygen-starved cells are unable to produce enough enzymes to fortify their cell walls and are thus more vulnerable to invasion. Disease microbes have no enzyme coating. When oxygen is introduced into the area, it attacks microbes without a coating and diseased cells with deficient cell wall enzymes. It oxidizes them, allowing them to be cleared from the body.

WHAT DEPLETES OXYGEN LEVELS IN THE BODY?

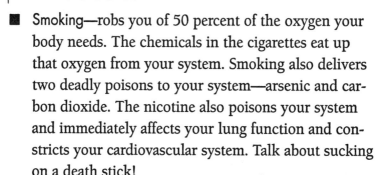

- Smoking—robs you of 50 percent of the oxygen your body needs. The chemicals in the cigarettes eat up that oxygen from your system. Smoking also delivers two deadly poisons to your system—arsenic and carbon dioxide. The nicotine also poisons your system and immediately affects your lung function and constricts your cardiovascular system. Talk about sucking on a death stick!
- Junk food—explored in chapter 2
- Shallow breathing
- Tap water (due to chlorine, fluoride, iodine)
- Food additives
- Sugars
- Fear, worry, depression
- Parasites
- Drugs
- Chemicals
- Lack of exercise
- Pollution/smog

These are only a few of the things that deplete oxygen levels in the body. Consider your lifestyle and see how you fit into some of these categories.

INCREASING YOUR BODY OXYGEN

- Consider your diet. Whether our bodies are sufficiently oxygenated to eliminate toxins and prevent disease depends greatly on our diets. I recommend eating God's way, the One Perfect Diet, the Levitical Diet! Calcium balance in the cells is critical in allowing oxygen into the body. Calcium absorption from digestion depends on Vitamin D, and most diets are deficient in it. Coenzyme Q10 and Vitamin C and E help the cell use its oxygen as well. Make a habit of eating five fresh fruits and vegetables a day. Not only will you get oxygen into your body, but you slash your risk of getting cancer by 30 percent, according to the American Cancer Society. A good liquid mineral supplement helps the body keep everything working in perfect harmony. Keeping your body in a healthy balance starts with a healthy diet, just as God designed it to do!

- Circulation of clean, oxygen-carrying blood is a basic requirement for healthy living. The first place to start is to daily practice deep-breathing techniques. This is the quickest way to increase oxygen levels. Starting right now, sit up straight so that you can get full lung capacity. Breathe in deeply through the nose and fill your lungs with oxygen, hold the breath for a few seconds, and slowly release the carbon monoxide out through the mouth. Do this several minutes each day! It is also excellent for relaxation.

- An ozone generator is a great investment and will give you rapid results.
- Good clean water is a must. I choose steam-distilled water and make certain that I get my minerals from my fresh fruits, veggies, and liquid minerals.
- Exercise is absolutely essential. You must exercise, even if you just start with walking in place. Start somewhere. Practice your deep-breathing techniques while you walk. Set your goal to exercise a little each day, 10-15 minutes, or 3-4 longer programs a week.
- Cut out all food chemicals. Read the labels on your foods, drinks, and even on your hair, skin, and personal items.
- Treat yourself once a week to an oxygen bath. The oxygen is absorbed through the pores, and oxygen levels are increased. Remember that your skin is the largest organ of your body. Oxygen bars are also now available in some areas. You have a seat, and they will hook you right up. I highly recommend my product, *Body Oxygen*™. The testimonials are endless of those who had deficient oxygen levels but were able to raise it to healthy levels after using it, as well as those just needing an extra pick-me-up. Keep in mind, though, that oxygen also makes you more alert and energetic, so be cautious when using it in the evening, unless you want to stay up past your usual bedtime.
- It is important to remember that fear, worry, and

depression all interfere with free breathing and thus reduce oxygen uptake. God has not given us a spirit of fear, but of power, love, and a sound mind (2 Timothy 1:7).

STILL DOUBTING?

The evidence is conclusive. Oxygen plays the primary role in health and well-being. When the body has sufficient oxygen, it is able to properly eliminate toxic wastes from the system. Natural immunity is enhanced when the system is not burdened with a heavy buildup of toxins. To allow your body to become under-oxygenated and remain in this condition can lead to severe health problems.

If you are still doubting, I found the 1997 Best Home Remedies of *Prevention Magazine* to be very interesting. It stated that deep breathing is the best solution for headaches, depression, cellulite, dropped bladder, and many other problems. I hope by now you understand why.

You should also consider an interesting study that I came across in Thibodeau's book on human anatomy, *Structure & Function of the Body,* which is used in medical schools all over the country. It was a study done in reference to athletes and military personnel that reported a number of athletes who improved their physical performance by a practice called Blood Doping. Here's how they did it. A few weeks before an important event, the athlete drew some blood. The RBCs (red blood cells that carry oxygen) were separated and frozen. Then just before the competition, the RBCs were thawed and injected back into the athlete.

The study showed that the increased hematocrit that results in the improved oxygen-carrying capacity of the blood improved the athlete's performance. This method was judged to be an unfair and unwise practice in athletes but has recently been investigated for use by the US armed services. They have reported that Blood Doping of soldiers just before combat could improve the soldiers' endurance for up to ten days.

What's interesting to me is that it is considered to be unfair in athletics. Is it that increased oxygen levels can make that great a change or advantage? You can answer that for yourself.

EXERCISE AND WATER

EXERCISE, NUTRITION, AND WEIGHT MANAGEMENT REPRESENT THE "BIG THREE" LIFESTYLE FACTORS THAT MOST PEOPLE LIST AS AFFECTING OUR HEALTH. I talk a lot in this book about how detoxifying your body is crucial to your health, and exercise gives that process a boost by improving the way oxygen is burned as well as how waste products are eliminated from the body tissues. Waste products are also removed through the increased sweat, weight is taken off, and weight control is made far easier because consistent exercise helps maintain your metabolism rate.

Nevertheless, the National Center for Chronic Disease Prevention and Health Promotion estimates that 60 percent of American adults exercise only once in a while, and 25 percent never exercise. Nearly half of American youths 12-21 years of age are not vigorously active on a regular basis. It's no surprise that every third person you meet is overweight. Sixty percent resort to medications to feel better, and 14 percent suffer from depression. Two out of five will die of heart disease.

Because so many Americans live sedentary lifestyles, women have acquired the "secretarial spread," and men have grown "love handles." Though those expressions are funny and cute, our out-of-proportion temples are nothing to laugh about.

According to a recent report of the Surgeon General on "Physical Activity and Health," *millions* of Americans suffer from illnesses that can be prevented or improved through regular physical activity. The numbers are mind-boggling. I sincerely hope, for your sake, that you are not among any of these categories.

- 13.5 million people have coronary heart disease.
- 1.5 million people suffer from a heart attack in a given year.
- 8 million people have Adult Onset (non-insulin-dependent) Diabetes.
- 95,000 people are newly diagnosed with colon cancer each year.
- 250,000 people suffer from hip fractures each year.
- 50 million people have high blood pressure.
- Over 60 million people (over a fourth of the population) are overweight.

THE BENEFITS OF EXERCISE

Regular physical activity (30 minutes of walking or raking leaves or 15 minutes of running) that is performed on most days of the week reduces the risk of developing or dying from some of the leading causes of illness and death in the United States. Regular physical activity improves health in the following ways:

- Reduces the risk of dying prematurely.
- Reduces the risk of dying prematurely from heart disease. It is hard to describe the extent of benefits that exercise brings to the cardiovascular system, but it's simple to explain why it happens. A good physical workout improves the strength of all the muscles in your body, particularly your heart muscle.
- Reduces the risk of developing diabetes, as it lowers the blood sugar level.
- Reduces the risk of developing high blood pressure.
- Helps reduce blood pressure in people who already have high blood pressure.
- Lowers triglyceride levels and raises HDL (good) blood cholesterol levels.
- Increases a person's sex drive.
- Reduces the risk of developing colon cancer. It also increases the motility of the colon and clears away constipation—just go for a walk in the morning and see how long it is before you're heading home for the bathroom!
- Helps control weight, develop lean muscle, and reduce body fat.
- Helps build and maintain healthy bones, muscles, and joints.
- Delays the development of osteoporosis.
- Helps older adults become stronger and better able to move about without falling.

- Increases the detoxification rate as well as the cellular turnover.
- Reduces symptoms of anxiety and depression and fosters improvements in mood and feelings of well-being. Exercise has the marvelous ability to remove the adrenaline that gets pumped into our bloodstream through stress, and thus it helps keep stress under control. Stress is a huge contributor to heart problems.

Physical activity also causes the release of endorphins, which in layman's terms are the body's natural feel-good hormones. Exercise is also helpful in normalizing women's hormone levels, and there is evidence to suggest that women who exercise regularly have significantly fewer problems with PMS, menopause, and breast cancer when compared to women who do not exercise.

IT'S TIME TO GET OFF THE COUCH!

Despite the grim statistics and the sedentary lifestyle most of us live, the human body was created by God for movement. Stu Mittleman, who is the author of *Slow Burn,* the marvelous book on running as a means of burning fat and unlocking the energy within, has said, "No other form of movement is as natural or as beneficial as running…. Our physiology is exquisitely designed for running and walking. It is only when we move in a bipedal motion—running or walking—that we can understand and appreciate the messages and innate wisdom our bodies offer. Our bodies are magnificently suited to moving in the form of walking and running. To engage in this motion brings us one step closer to what we are."

I am not suggesting that you need to jump out of your chair and commit yourself to spending hours on end at the local gym, but I am a proponent of breaking the lethargy syndrome that seems to bind so many people I meet. You were not designed by God to come home at the end of the day and plop down in front of the television for the last hours of the day after having sat at a desk for 8+ hours. Your body was not made for inactivity while you pour in the calories with a poor diet. It's a recipe for disaster.

Check out the following chart from the *Dietary Guidelines for Americans* that compares the number of calories your body burns during one hour of various activities. These statistics are based on a healthy man of 175 pounds and a healthy woman of 140 pounds.

Activity	Calories Used Per Hour	
	Man	Woman
Sitting quietly	100	80
Standing quietly	120	95
Light activity:	300	240
Cleaning house		
Office work		
Playing baseball/golf		
Moderate activity:	460	370
Walking briskly (3.5 mph)		
Cycling (5.5 mph)		
Gardening, Dancing		
Playing basketball		
Strenuous activity:	730	580

Jogging (9 min. mile)		
Playing football		
Swimming		
Very strenuous activity	920	740
Running (7 min. mile)		
Racquetball		
Skiing		

WHERE TO START?

There are countless ways to begin exercising. Any type of exercise is better than none. You do not have to become an athlete. Take your spouse's hand and head out the door for a comfortable walk, burn some calories, and perhaps put a little spark of romance in your day. Depending on the distance to your job, consider walking. Park your car at the farthest end from the store entrance and take a little stroll before going inside. Something as simple as climbing five flights of stairs every day will significantly lower your risk of heart disease. Every step you walk or run burns calories.

There are any number of exercise choices available to you. There's fast walking, jogging, cycling, swimming, weight-lifting, calisthenics, dance, hiking, skating, tennis, basketball, aerobics, martial arts, rollerblading, and on and on. Some find that a membership at a health club keeps them motivated as well as provides all the equipment they like to use, others prefer to set up a home gym, while others stick more with an aerobic program that requires little or no equipment.

Let's face it, though—there's no shortage of exercise

choices or ways to do those exercises. The question is whether we make health and fitness a priority in our lives.

BEFORE YOU START

- If you are over 40, in poor health, have risk factors for coronary artery disease, high blood pressure, or diabetes, shortness of breath, or heart irregularity, a treadmill test is highly recommended. A physician or exercise specialist can provide this test. It is a test that checks blood pressure and uses an electrocardiogram to monitor heart performance. Better to be safe than sorry.

- Think about your goals. Setting and meeting short- and long-term goals is a tremendous encouragement to keep developing and maintaining an exercise program. Your goal might be to achieve a target heart rate each day or to walk a certain distance, but having something to shoot at will keep you focused.

- Whatever exercise you choose, get the right equipment to help you facilitate that exercise. For instance, if you are going to walk or run, go to a shoe store that specializes in running and talk with trained personnel who know what you'll need. Saving $20 or $30 on a cheaper pair of shoes that you can "live with" isn't worth it. Spend the time and make sure you start well. Also, make certain that you have the right fitting clothes for the exercise. Choose bright colors for safety reasons. Again, you don't need to spend a fortune on fancy clothes, but you need the right clothes.

- If you are really out of shape, begin your physical

activity program with short sessions (5-10 minutes) of physical activity and gradually build up to the desired level of activity (30 minutes). As long as you're keeping active, you're becoming fitter without even realizing it. You don't have to run marathons for your health to reap significant benefits. You just need to be consistent.

■ Keep in mind that physical activity does not need to be strenuous to achieve health benefits. The same moderate amount of activity can be obtained in longer sessions of moderately intense activities (such as 30 minutes of brisk walking) as in shorter sessions of more strenuous activities (such as 15-20 minutes of jogging). Additional health benefits can be gained through greater amounts of physical activity. Adults who maintain a regular routine of physical activity that is of longer duration or of greater intensity are likely to derive greater benefit. However, because risk of injury also increases with greater amounts of activity, care should be taken to avoid excessive amounts.

■ Consider weather conditions. Excessive heat or cold must be seriously considered. Never put yourself at risk.

■ Drink water—before, during, and after exercise, especially during warm weather. Replacing water lost by sweating is crucial.

■ Don't overdo it. Pushing too hard can lead to damage.

■ Check with a doctor immediately if you ever have symptoms such as chest pain or pressure, heart irregularity, or unusual shortness of breath.

STRETCHING

Before starting to exercise, spend five to ten minutes doing warm-up stretching exercises, no matter how intense your workout is going to be. To properly stretch your muscles lessens the likelihood of any muscles being damaged.

It is also good to spend the last five minutes of your exercise program doing the same stretching exercises to increase your flexibility. This will also help your heart rate and muscles return to normal as well as help your body to cool down.

Here are three stretches that I recommend. Do each of the warm-up activities three times.

- **Hamstring stretch.** The hamstrings are the big muscles in the back of your thigh. Place one foot on a chair, and the other about 18 inches away. Keep your back straight and lean your arms on the bent knee and gradually lean forward until you feel the upper part of the straight leg being stretched. Hold it for a count of 20, and then repeat with the other leg.

- **Quadriceps stretch.** The quadriceps muscle is on the front of your thighs. Place your left hand against a wall for balance. While standing straight, bend your right knee, bringing your foot up and back, while reaching back with your left hand to grasp the right foot. Avoid straightening the left knee completely. Grab your right ankle with your right hand and pull toward your buttocks for a count of 20. Then repeat with the other leg.

- Upper body stretch. Standing in an upright position and clasping your hands behind your back, make sure your elbows remain straight. Pull your shoulders back, and then bend forward, lifting your arms above your head, elbows still straight and hands clasped. Stand straight again and, holding your clasped hands away from your buttock and keeping your elbows straight, twist your upper body to the right and to the left twice.

WALKING IS A WISE CHOICE

I recommend that you consider walking as a great starting point for exercise. It brings all the health benefits listed previously, and it is a very doable exercise. Recent studies have shown that a brisk walk provides strenuous enough exercise for cardiovascular training in most adults. And unlike running, it puts little strain on your knees and legs.

The results of a twelve-year study of the exercise habits and mortality rates of 17,000 Harvard alumni were recently released. It found that men who walked a lot and were otherwise physically active lived longer. Also, life expectancy improved steadily as exercise increased, starting at 500 calories spent per week, and continuing up to 3,500 calories per week. Exercising more than that was counterproductive.

PACE YOURSELF

As you set goals for how long you are going to exercise, keep in mind that it's okay to be a bit out of breath, but not so much that you can't talk. Pace your workout so that you push without overdoing it. If you are still tired an hour after the exercise, you should back off a bit and build up slower.

If you prefer to be more scientific about it, measure your heart rate by taking your pulse. Aim for a heart rate between 70 and 80 percent of the maximum for your age group. If you need to lose weight, you can achieve the greatest loss if you aim for about 60 percent of your maximum heart rate and exercise for 45-60 minutes three to five times a week.

Age	70-80% of Max Rate	60% of Max Rate
20	140-160	120
30	133-152	114
40	126-144	108
50	119-136	102
60	112-128	96
70	105-120	90

PRACTICAL EXERCISE TIPS

1. Schedule exercise into your family life. Write it in as if it's an important meeting—one that can't be missed or rescheduled.

2. Start where you are. No matter what physical shape you are currently in, you can begin some sort of exercise program. If you can't get out of the house to walk, start by walking in place. Then, increase slowly! Every little bit helps. Even if you are in a wheelchair, start with lifting three-pound dumbbells. Just do it!

3. Use what you have! You don't have to buy an expensive club membership to start exercising. You can walk or ride your bike for free! If you desire exercise instruction, check out a book or an instructional video at your local library.

4. **Exercise consistently.** Exercise at least three times a week for 20-30 minutes. You will be amazed at how this will help to cut your cravings and give you more energy immediately. The longevity you will receive from your 90-minute investment will serve you well.

5. **Get an exercise buddy.** If you have trouble staying motivated, then get a partner to help you keep your commitment. If you have an exercise buddy, you'll be more likely to show up for exercise times. Plus, it's a lot of fun to share workouts with a friend.

6. **Improvise!** Maybe you don't have expensive weights or elaborate exercise equipment in your home, but you do have green bean cans and stairs. Well, use a green bean can in each hand for dumbbells, and use your stairs as a pseudo stair-stepping machine. Your body won't know the difference—trust me!

7. **Take advantage of everyday activities.** Take the stairs instead of the elevator at work. Do this every time you go somewhere, and you'll discover how much these little changes make for big results.

8. **Make the most of waiting.** If you have to wait for a long document to print (and you have a private office), do a few squats or knee lunges while waiting. If you're not dressed for calisthenics, do some deep breathing and stretching.

WATER! WATER! WATER! YOU CAN'T GET TOO MUCH

Water, water, water! You can't get enough! Did you

know that you are 65-70 percent water? Even your bones are 10 percent water.

Without water, there can be no life. This is because all the life processes—from taking in food to getting rid of wastes—require water. Water maintains homeostasis, or balance, in the cells, where everything is working correctly. Watery solutions help dissolve nutrients and carry them to all parts of your body. Through chemical reactions that can only take place in a watery solution, your system turns nutrients into energy or into materials it needs to grow to repair cells. Water is used for every enzyme process that governs the nerve chemicals, and therefore every thought and action, every chemical process, and therefore every function in the body.

Every living thing must keep its water supply near normal or it will die. Human beings can live without food for months, but they can live without water for only about a week. If the body loses more than 20 percent of its normal water content, a person will die painfully.

It should go without saying that you need to drink a lot of water. But as a whole, people are not replenishing the very element God put in them. Dehydration can be the cause of constipation, fatigue, lung and urinary infections, creaking and stiff joints, dizziness, headaches, hunger, and dry skin conditions.

You should be drinking at least half your body weight in ounces of water. For example, if you weigh 150 pounds, you should drink at least 75 ounces (a little more than one half a gallon) of water per day. Do some quick math and determine how much water you should be drinking each day. So the standard daily guideline of eight 8-ounce glasses each day may not be enough agua for you. This is particularly true if you are in hot weather or exercising or sweating for whatever reason.

Drinks that contain alcohol and caffeine, such as coffee, teas, or soft drinks, do not count the same volume as water, because they increase the loss of water from the body in urine. This leaves the body dehydrated. Replace these drinks with herb and fruit teas or coffee substitutes made with barley or rye, chicory, or dandelion. Substitute diluted fruit juices or herbal cocktail drinks for alcoholic drinks.

BENEFITS OF WATER

Sparkling pure water with ice and a slice of lemon— think of these benefits:

- Flushes the kidneys and liver, enabling them to remove toxins from your body. You may have to urinate more, but that's a good thing. The bladder will be dumping out unwanted substances.
- Reduces feelings of hunger. You may be mistaking hunger pangs for thirst signals.
- Maintains energy levels. A 2 percent loss of water surrounding the cells of the body can lead to a loss of energy by up to 20 percent.
- Controls the temperature of the body and eliminates toxins through sweat.
- Increases the efficiency of your immune system.

- Keeps your skin looking good and feeling soft.
- Reduces the risk of developing kidney stones and gallstones.
- Reduces the risk of developing headaches.
- Keeps your brain active. Dehydration may contribute to memory loss and senility.

WHY I BELIEVE IN STEAM-DISTILLED WATER

I constantly stress the importance of drinking steam-distilled water. I know there is controversy over steam distilled, but I think it's the best water for your body. Some medical authorities think it throws off our biochemical/ electrical balance and prefer regular, purified water. Obviously, I don't agree.

I explain my reasoning with a simple example. When you buy water for an iron, you always buy steam distilled, right? If you use tap water, your iron will spat and sputter, trying to filter out all the chemicals contained in tap water (chlorine, fluoride, and iodine). And if you continue using tap water, soon there will be so much buildup that you will not be able to use your iron.

On the other hand, by using distilled water, everything flows freely, and the iron remains in perfect working order for years. Think of your body as though it is an iron. Because of its lack of minerals and flat molecular structure, distilled water draws other particles (nutrients and toxins) to it, which actually pulls out the toxins that build up in the body. Yes, you urinate more, but it's simply the bladder dumping more as the water pulls out unwanted substances. That's a good thing.

Here's another benefit of drinking distilled water. It will help rid your body of those awful cravings—the ones that make you stop at a convenience store to buy a snack you know isn't good for you. As the water flushes out your system, it cleanses the remainder of that junk food you've been consuming. Remember the last food that you ate will be the next food you crave. So if you are loading up with junk, you will continue craving it if you do not get it flushed out of your system.

Need more reasons to drink steam-distilled water? Well, it has a pH level of 7.0, meaning it will help bring up your pH so that you are not acidic, but more on the alkaline side. Doctors and scientists agree that by keeping the body more alkaline, you are more likely to remain free from disease.

CLEANSE YOUR SYSTEM OF THE BAD STUFF

"Is not this the kind of fasting I have chosen: to loose the chains of injustice and untie the cords of the yoke, to set the oppressed free and break every yoke? Is it not to share your food with the hungry and to provide the poor wanderer with shelter—when you see the naked, to clothe him, and not to turn away from your own flesh and blood? Then your light will break forth like the dawn, and your healing will quickly appear, then your righteousness will go before you, and the glory of the Lord will be your rear guard."

ISAIAH 58:6-8

CANDIDA ALBICANS

WHAT IS CANDIDA ALBICANS?

CANDIDA ALBICANS IS A PARASITIC YEASTLIKE FUNGUS THAT EXISTS NATURALLY IN THE BODY AND USUALLY CAUSES NO BAD EFFECTS. It mainly inhabits the digestive tract but can spread to other parts of the body such as the esophagus, mouth, throat, genital area, and even the lungs in severe cases. In a normal healthy body, these harmless parasites coexist in small colonies along with the other bacteria found in our digestive system.

The immune system and the "friendly" bacteria in our intestines (*Bifidobacteria bifidum* and *Lactobacillus acidophilus*) keep *Candida* overgrowth under control most of the time in a healthy body. These bacteria and others make up the normal bacterial population of our gastrointestinal tract and are often referred to as "GI microflora." They exist in a symbiotic relationship with us and are essential for maintaining healthy intestines and resisting infections. However, when an imbalance occurs in the natural bacterial environment, which can be caused by a variety of factors, then the *Candida Albicans* organisms begin to grow at a rapid rate and spread and infect the body tissues.

These "colonies" of the *Candida Albicans* are anaerobic organisms (existing in the absence of oxygen), and when they occur in large numbers, they can release their toxic waste directly into the bloodstream, which can cause a number of symptoms. It is estimated that over 90 percent of the U.S. population has some degree of *Candida* overgrowth in their bodies.

THE CAUSES OF CANDIDA ALBICANS

Why does this yeast, which is normally harmless, tend to grow out of control? There are a number of factors that reduce our natural resistance and contribute to *Candidiasis,* an overgrowth of *Candida.* These causes include:

1. Extended use of antibiotics. The prevalence that we now see with the *Candida* problem in large part can be attributed to the widespread use of broad-spectrum antibiotics that are prescribed for all kinds of infections. They are especially harmful because they destroy not only the disease-causing bacteria but also the "friendly" bacteria that help to control the *Candida* bacteria. As a result, an imbalance occurs in the pH levels of our intestines, which in turn stimulates the growth of the *Candida.*

The Latin definition of a *biotic* is *life.* So an antibiotic is anti-life, and a probiotic is pro-life.

2. Oral contraceptives. These types of drugs cause a hormone imbalance, which also favors the growth of *Candida.*

3. Low levels of acidophilus and bifidus bacteria in the colon. When these "friendly" bacteria levels are reduced, then the *Candida* bacteria have free reign to grow out of control.

4. Improper diets. The average American diet is also a cause for *Candida.* A lot of the food we consume is overprocessed,

high in refined sugar and carbohydrates, and low in fiber. It is no wonder that we have a problem with yeast infections when you consider all the fast-food we eat in our fast-paced society. Our lifestyles have drastically affected our eating habits. According to a *Journal of American Medical Association* article in 1977, this kind of diet results in fewer "friendly" bacteria in our gastrointestinal tract. Those conditions then favor the onset of *Candidiasis*.

5. Chemicals. It is no secret that since the turn of the twentieth century we have introduced thousands of chemicals into our environment. We have paid a price in terms of our health because prolonged exposure to many of them over the years has had a host of adverse effects on our health. A number of those chemicals have entered our food chains through growth hormones given to livestock or by chemicals used in the feed to prevent disease. Other chemicals and pollutants such as fertilizers have leached off thousands of farms into rivers and steams, thus contaminating fish. It is a sad commentary on the state of our environment that in some states information on contaminated streams and rivers is given when fishing licenses are issued. Even chemicals such as chlorine found in our drinking water can have an effect on the growth of *Candida Albicans*.

It can be one of these causes or a combination of all of them to different degrees that can throw our bodies out of balance. The human body was "fearfully and wonderfully made," but it has its limits also. When we cross those limits, and a serious flare-up of *Candidiasis* occurs, then we may experience a variety of alarming symptoms.

THE SYMPTOMS OF CANDIDA ALBICANS

Yeast infections can occur in anybody at any age, but they are more prevalent in women. When our body systems become imbalanced, then a yeast overgrowth can occur. It is possible for someone to have a problem for a while before they manifest symptoms.

Candida Albicans can exist in two forms: yeast and fungal. Serious health problems can develop when it changes its anatomy to a fungal form. In that state, the organisms produce rhizoids (very long rootlike structures) that penetrate the mucous lining of the intestine. These rhizoids leave tiny holes that break down the natural barrier between the intestines and the circulatory system and allow toxins, bacteria, yeast, and even small undigested food particles direct access to the bloodstream. Once these toxins enter the bloodstream, they can travel throughout the entire body and produce a number of adverse symptoms that further weaken the immune system. These include:

- constipation
- diarrhea
- colitis
- abdominal pain
- headaches
- bad breath
- rectal itching
- impotence
- memory loss
- mood swings
- prostatitis
- canker sores
- persistent heartburn
- muscle and joint pain
- sore throat
- congestion
- nagging cough
- numbness in the face or extremities
- tingling sensations

- acne
- night sweats
- severe itching
- clogged sinuses
- PMS
- burning tongue
- white spots on the tongue and in the mouth
- vaginitis
- kidney and bladder infections
- arthritis
- depression
- hyperactivity
- hypothyroidism
- adrenal problems
- Jock itch
- athlete's foot
- even diabetes
- immune weakness
- poor digestion
- chronic fatigue
- bloating
- gas
- poor elimination
- sugar and carbohydrate cravings
- head pain
- brain fog
- female issues
- skin rashes
- cold hands or feet

Symptoms often worsen in damp and/or moldy places, and after consumption of foods containing sugar and/or yeast, as well as after a round of antibiotics. Because this disorder is oftentimes misdiagnosed, many individual symptoms are treated, but the sufferer from *Candida Albicans* often never gets to the root of the problem.

People who have been battling any chronic symptoms listed above without relief should explore the possibility of *Candida* overgrowth and take the necessary steps to alleviate this condition. The following is one way to determine if you have a problem with *Candida*.

CANDIDA ALBICANS SELF-TEST ✍

In order to properly understand and diagnose whether you have a problem with *Candida Albicans,* it is necessary to take a look at your personal medical history and administer a *Candida* questionnaire. The information will then help determine what may have promoted to the *Candida* growth in the first place. Circle the points below that apply to you and then add the total at the end of the section.

The diagnosis of *Candida Albicans* is somewhat controversial, as the scientific proof is not conclusive. If your test score is high, and you think you have this problem, you may wish to consult a licensed medical professional. Information in this book, including comments on medical treatments, is not intended as medical advice. It should be evaluated critically and should not take the place of medical advice from a licensed healthcare professional.

PERSONAL HISTORY QUESTIONNAIRE ✍

1. During your lifetime, have you taken any antibiotics or tetracyclines (symycin, Panmycin, Vibramycin, Monicin, etc.) for acne or other conditions for more than one month?   25 pts.
2. Have you taken a broad-spectrum antibiotic for more than 2 months or 4 or more times in a 1-year period? These could include any antibiotics taken for respiratory, urinary, or other infections.   20 pts.

3. Have you taken a broad-spectrum antibiotic even for a single course? These antibiotics include ampicillin, amoxicillin, Keflex, etc.   6 pts.

4. Have you ever had problems with persistent Prostatitis, vaginitis, or other problems with your reproductive organs?   25 pts.

5. Women—Have you been pregnant?
   2 or more times?   5 pts.
   1 time?   3 pts.

6. Women—Have you taken birth control pills?
   More than 2 years?   15 pts.
   More than 6 months?   8 pts.

7. If you were NOT breast-fed as an infant.   9 pts.

8. Have you taken any cortisone-type drugs (Prednisone, Decadron, etc.)?   15 pts.

9. Are you sensitive to and bothered by exposure to perfumes, insecticides, or other chemical odors . . .   20 pts.
   Do you have moderate to severe symptoms?   20 pts.
   Mild symptoms?   5 pts.

10. Does tobacco smoke bother you?   10 pts.

11. Are your symptoms worse on damp, muggy days or in moldy places?   20 pts.

12. If you have had chronic fungus infections of the skin or nails (including athlete's foot, ringworm, jock itch), have the infections been . . .
   Severe or persistent?   20 pts.
   Mild to moderate?   10 pts.

13. Do you crave sugar (chocolate, ice cream,

candy, cookies, etc.)? | 10 pts.

14. Do you crave carbohydrates (bread, bread, and more bread)? | 10 pts.

15. Do you crave alcoholic beverages? | 10 pts.

16. Have you drunk or do you drink chlorinated water (city or tap)? | 20 pts.

TOTAL _____

SCORE YOUR SYMPTOMS

For each of your symptoms, enter the corresponding number in the point score column.

No symptoms 0
Occasional or mild 3
Frequent or moderately severe 6
Severe and/or disabling 9

SYMPTOMS	POINTS
1. Constipation	9
2. Diarrhea	9
3. Bloating
4. Fatigue or lethargy	6
5. Feeling drained	6
6. Poor memory
7. Difficulty focusing/brain fog	6
8. Feeling moody or despaired
9. Numbness, burning, or tingling	6
10. Muscle aches	6
11. Nasal congestion or discharge	6
12. Pain and/or swelling in the joints	3

13. Abdominal pain   *6*
14. Spots in front of the eyes   *6*
15. Erratic vision   *6*
16. Cold hands and/or feet   *6*
17. Women—endometriosis   _____
18. Women—menstrual irregularities   _____
19. Women—premenstrual tension   _____
20. Women—vaginal discharge   _____
21. Women—persistent vaginal
    burning or itching   *3*
22. Men—prostatitis   _____
23. Men—impotence   _____
24. Loss of sexual desire   _____
25. Low blood sugar   _____
26. Anger or frustration
27. Dry patchy skin   *3*
TOTAL   *81*

CANDIDA SELF-TEST

For each of your symptoms, enter the appropriate figure in the point score column.

No symptoms .0
Occasional or mild 3
Frequent or moderately severe 6
Severe and/or disabling 9

1. Heartburn   *3*
2. Indigestion   *6*
3. Belching and intestinal gas   *6*

4. Drowsiness   6

5. Itching   6

6. Rashes   0

7. Irritability or jitters   3

8. Uncoordinated   6

9. Inability to concentrate   3

10. Frequent mood swings   3

11. Postnasal drip   —

12. Nasal itching   —

13. Failing vision   3

14. Burning or tearing of the eyes   3

15. Recurrent infections or fluid in the ears   6

16. Ear pain or deafness   6

17. Headaches   3

18. Dizziness/loss of balance   3

19. Pressure above the ears—your head feels
as though it is swelling   3

20. Mucus in the stools   3

21. Hemorrhoids   6

22. Dry mouth   6

23. Rash or blisters in the mouth   —

24. Bad breath   —

25. Sore or dry throat   6

26. Cough   3

27. Pain or tightness in the chest   —

28. Wheezing or shortness of breath   6

29. Urinary urgency or frequency   6

30. Burning during urination   3

TOTAL   —

CANDIDA SELF-ANALYSIS RESULTS

Total Score from Section 1   _____
Total Score from Section 2   _____
Total Score from Section 3   _____
TOTAL SCORE   _____

If your score is at least:	Your symptoms are:
180 Women / 140 Men	Almost certainly yeast connected
120 Women / 90 Men	Probably yeast connected
60 Women / 40 Men	Possibly yeast connected

If your score is less than:	
60 Women / 40 Men	Probably not yeast connected

If you scored below 60 for women or 40 for men, WAY TO GO! You are probably not plagued with the symptoms of *Candida Albicans*. You are obviously following a very healthy lifestyle, and you deserve a huge pat on the back! However, if your score was above 60 for women or 40 for men, you may want to consider looking into a means to get the *Candida* overgrowth under control.

TREATMENT OF CANDIDA ALBICANS

If you are going to rid your body of *Candida* successfully, then you are going to have to make changes in your lifestyle. The most important first step to overcoming this infection will be changing your diet. Our goal is to rid the body of the yeast infection and restore the normal flora balance in our intestines so that our body can heal itself. A clean colon is essential if we are going to succeed against a severe case of *Candida Albicans*. See chapter 7 on fasting for the importance of enemas for cleansing the body of toxins. It is extremely important that you remove old impacted fecal matter and excess mucous that is adhering to the inner wall of your intestinal walls. Because the organisms thrive in those materials that are warm, putrid, and lacking in oxygen, it is necessary to thoroughly cleanse your intestines and then adapt radical changes to the way you eat in order to treat the problem effectively. The following are recommendations to rid the body and starve out the *Candida*:

DO'S

- Change toothbrushes every 30 days, as mold and fungus will tend to grow over prolonged use. Daily rinse your toothbrush with a good *food grade* hydrogen peroxide to kill bacteria on the brush as well as in the mouth. After rinsing the toothbrush with 3 percent hydrogen peroxide, do not wash off with tap water, apply toothpaste directly to brush.
- Pau d'arco tea contains an antibacterial agent and can be used up to six times a day until symptoms subside. Alternating with Clove tea is an excellent way to kill the fungus. These also store well in the fridge. So you can make them ahead and seal for future use.
- Use only steam-distilled water when cooking. And you should be drinking half your weight in ounces of steam-distilled water to eliminate chemical contaminants. For instance, if you weigh 128 pounds, you

should drink 64 ounces or a half a gallon spaced throughout the day.

- Eat a cup of oat bran daily to speed up elimination.
- Eat fresh and raw vegetables, which will help to restore the normal intestinal flora in your body. Bake, broil, or steam your vegetables.
- If you are suffering with a yeast infection or jock itch, clean genital area morning and evening with Tea Tree oil. Dilute 8 ounces warm distilled water with 8 drops Tea Tree oil. Clean with cloth.
- Eat yogurt (no Aspartame®) daily, as much as possible, with live active cultures that are documented on the label! These help to restore the natural "friendly" bacteria to your gastrointestinal tract.
- Women, douching 2-3 times per week with H_2O_2 mixture of 1 ounce 3 percent food grade hydrogen peroxide to 11 ounces distilled water may be helpful.
- Kyolic® garlic 2 capsules, 3 times per day are very helpful, and a good B-Complex is an excellent addition. Capricin®, (Cayenne pepper) 4 capsules, 3 times per day.
- Natren Probiotics, daily. It creates a good terrain for aerobic bacteria (good bacteria) to live and thrive in, also use,
- *Body Oxygen*™ 2-3 times per day and,
- *Oxygen Bath*™ 2-3 per week.
- Lastly, take a good supplement that attacks the *Candida*.

DON'TS

- Avoid taking antibiotics unless absolutely necessary. Remember to eat plenty of yogurt if you do take a round of antibiotics that has been prescribed by a physician.

- Avoid oral contraceptives and cortisone products, which work against the effectiveness of this regime and should be discussed with your health care professional.

- Avoid aged cheeses, alcohol, chocolate, dried fruits, fermented foods, all grains containing gluten, pork, honey, nut butters, pickles, raw mushrooms, soy sauce, sprouts, sugars of all forms, soft drinks, vinegar, and all yeast products.

- Avoid citrus and acid fruits (orange, grapefruit, tomatoes, pineapple, and limes) until all signs of *Candida* are gone for 3 months.

- Avoid all meats that have been treated with hormones or chemicals.

- Avoid saturated fats.

CONCLUSION

If left untreated, *Candida Albicans* can become a dangerous infection that will spread and weaken the body's immune system to fight off disease. Because I believe in the body's amazing ability to heal itself when we follow the guidelines God has given us, I strongly suggest using this natural approach to remove this yeastlike fungus from your body. By eliminating it from your system, it will especially take the stress off of your immune system.

There may be some cases that are so severe they require special treatment from a licensed health care professional. There are certain drugs that have been used by some to treat severe cases of *Candida Albicans*. Please consult a medical doctor if the need arises.

By taking the steps to rid your body of an overgrowth of *Candida Albicans*, you will be restoring health to your body, allowing it to function the way God intended. You will be amazed at the release of new energy you will experience as you rid your body of the toxins that have been poisoning it. Remember, you can do it!

DETOXIFICATION

DETOXIFICATION IS A CLEANSING PROCESS THAT IS GOING ON INSIDE YOUR BODY EVERY SECOND OF YOUR LIFE. If your body fails to eliminate its toxins daily, eventually you will die an earlier death than you should have. Our purpose here is to explore ways you can help this process that is so essential to rejuvenating the body and helping you feel great all the time. You can improve the quality of your life as well as the length of your life by following the suggestions I set forth in this chapter.

Fasting is one method of detoxification to which I have devoted the entirety of chapter 7. I consider it the most effective and practical and quickest way to cleanse your system. Yet I recognize that it is a more extreme form. There are many ways to detoxify, some of which we will consider in this chapter.

No one escapes toxins in this world. A toxin describes the chemicals in your body that have not been "detoxed" (made harmless). Toxicity occurs on two primary levels. First, toxins are taken in from our environment through the air we breathe, the food and water we consume, and through physical contact with them—environmental pollutants, food additives, and chemicals being the major ones. The majority of allergens and drugs and also mercury fillings in the teeth can create toxic elements in the body.

Second, your body produces toxins naturally all the time. Biochemical, cellular, and bodily activities generate waste substances that need to be eliminated. Free radicals, for instance, are biochemical toxins. When these are not removed, they can cause tissues and cells to become irritated or inflamed, blocking normal functions on a cellular, organ, and whole-body level. Yeasts, intestinal bacteria, foreign bacteria, and parasites produce metabolic waste products that we must process and eliminate from our bodies. Even stress creates a toxic state, if we allow it to dominate our mind and emotions.

Your body was designed by God to eliminate toxins, but over time these chemicals can build up in your system and overwhelm your ability to remove them. Or you yourself might be overpowering your system by the amount of toxins you are taking in physically, emotionally, or spiritually. Some drugs and many pesticides produce immediate, dramatic toxic symptoms. Others take a long time to develop into a manifest disease, such as asbestos exposure that invisibly leads to lung cancer. It is no surprise that toxicity diseases such as cardiovascular disease and cancer have increased as our world has become more toxic. Many skin problems, allergies, arthritis, and obesity are others. In addition, a wide range of less frightening symptoms, such as headaches, fatigue, pains, coughs, constipation, gastrointestinal problems, and problems from immune weakness, can all be related to toxicity.

Your Body Is a Total System

You were given five central systems that work together moment by moment to eliminate toxins. It is your responsibility to maintain their health. These systems include the *respiratory*—lungs, bronchial tubes, throat, sinuses, and nose; *gastrointestinal*—liver, gallbladder, colon, and whole GI tract; *urinary*—kidneys, bladder, and urethra; *skin and dermal*—sweat and sebaceous glands and tears; and *lymphatic*—lymph channels and lymph nodes.

As we saw in chapter 1, the liver filters out foreign substances and wastes from the blood, metabolically altering the toxins and making them easier for the organs to eliminate and less harmful to the body. It also dumps wastes through the bile into the intestines, where much waste is eliminated. The kidneys filter wastes from the blood into the urine, while the lungs remove volatile gases as we breathe. We also clear heavy metals through sweating. Our sinuses and skin may also be accessory elimination organs whereby excess mucus or toxins can be released, as with sinus congestion or skin rashes.

A detoxification program is designed to safely and gently enhance your body's own natural processes. It can be done at several levels and refers to many different programs that cleanse the body of toxins. Anything that promotes elimination can be said to help us detoxify. Drinking more water will usually help you eliminate more toxins. Eating more fruits and vegetables—the high-water-content, cleansing foods—and less meat and dairy products creates less congestion and more elimination. Some programs are directed toward specific organs, such as the liver or kidneys or skin. The secret to great health and feeling great is to combine these detoxification programs into a lifestyle program that works for you. The goal is to become so aware of your body that you know when things are right and instinctively know what you need. It can happen!

Is it possible to go overboard on detoxifying? Certainly, and I see it occasionally. Some people go to extremes with fasting, laxatives, enemas, colonics, diuretics, and exercise, and begin to lose essential nutrients from their body. Some people push it to the point where they experience dangerous protein or vitamin-mineral deficiencies, even becoming paranoid to the extent of bondage! But in America, the vast percentage of our health concerns result from the opposite of going overboard on detoxifying.

It is proven that many common serious and chronic diseases may be diminished or eliminated by a program of cleansing. People with addictions to any substance regularly benefit from detoxification programs, even if it is only the temporary avoidance of the addictive agent or agents. You will feel better when your system gets rid of the unchanged or partially changed toxins that cause negative symptoms. Your immune system will be strengthened in its relentless battle against infections, and you may also reduce the risk of developing cancer. Many of the poisons (toxins) that we take in or make are stored in the fatty tissues. Obesity is almost always associated with toxicity. When we lose weight, we reduce our fat and thereby our toxic load.

WHAT ARE YOU EATING?

Step #1—*start eating right*. If you cut your toxic intake, you cut your need for cleansing. I've heard it said that a Twinkie has a shelf life of twenty years. What does that say about the synthetic chemicals that get into our systems? If you don't correct a bad diet, you drastically reduce the effectiveness of any other cleansing methods you use. I have one entire chapter dedicated to my preference in detoxification diets, which is called the Levitical Diet. I favor it because it is well balanced and proven to have been effective for thousands of years.

Detoxification diets help the body eliminate toxins in many ways. They generally eliminate the foods that commonly trigger problems with digestion and elimination. Foods such as wheat and dairy products are often the cause of allergies. Refined, processed, and junk foods are also out for any detoxification program to work. Sugar is drastically cut because of its "empty calories" and tendency to produce hypoglycemia as well as feed cancer cells. Meats are cut back or eliminated because they may contain hormones, antibiotics, and require many enzymes for digestion.

Natural vegetarian diets are cleansing and bring the body several benefits. You get plenty of fiber to stimulate the bowels as well as generous amounts of vitamins to feed and nourish all the eliminative organs. They also include a valuable source of enzymes, since most vegetarian diets are eaten raw. However, even vegetarians can be very off balance due to a lack of good protein and essential salts.

My favorite diet is about 70 percent fruits, vegetables, nuts, and grains; 25 percent cold-water fish and hormone-free chicken; and about 3-5 percent hormone-free red meat. Once again, by knowing your body, you will know what you need.

Whatever diet you choose, *it must be balanced.* If you have any questions regarding your diet, consult a professional nutritionist, Naturopath, or physician. I have included a number of general tips on eating and food (see pages 151) that you will find helpful.

WHAT ARE YOU DRINKING?

In chapter 4, I deal extensively with the importance of water in any type of detoxification program. Your body does not have a better detoxifying friend than water. To adequately help dilute and eliminate toxin accumulations from your body, I recommend that you drink half your body weight in ounces of steam-distilled water every day. From the vital flushing of the kidneys and liver to keeping your skin looking good and feeling soft, the benefits are universal. I suggest you drink water 30-60 minutes before each meal and even at night to help flush toxins during your body's natural elimination time.

FROM START TO FINISH

While it's a subject most of us prefer not to discuss, cleansing the bowels consistently is a vital key to good health. Your bowels should move like a newborn's, many times a day. One movement now and then is dangerous, but can be changed. When the bowels slow down, the bad news begins. First, there is an increase of bad bacteria in the small intestine and putrefaction in the large intestine. The battle ensues when the bad bacteria weaken your immune system (which is located in the small intestine) and can result in digestive complications. When only partly digested proteins and bacterial toxins cross the intestinal wall, they can cause allergies.

Untreated, it gets ugly. The walls of the bowels become weak and deformed, as with diverticulitis, and hard crusts cover the intestinal walls and restrict movement within the bowels. In severe cases, the products of putrefaction cross the weakened walls of the large intestine and enter the bloodstream. The whole body may become poisoned, and it is possible to seriously damage your body. Enemas and colonics may be needed to break up and cleanse the bowel encrustations.

Reabsorbed toxins are carried back to the liver for recycling and elimination, causing stress to the liver, which then produces extra bile salts that are linked to increased cholesterol levels. Also, when the bowels constipate and toxin levels increase, the bad bacteria grow to outnumber the normal flora and cause dysbiosis. Every part of your nervous system may be affected, and sometimes the heart or brain takes the brunt of the damage.

The easiest way to correct these intestinal problems is a diet of predominately raw foods. A high-quality fiber diet of fresh fruits and vegetables gets the bowels moving and strengthens the bowel walls. You may want to add extra fiber by drinking a glass of water (juice) with psyllium husk powder or another herbal laxative or 1/2 cup of oat bran daily to speed up the process. But it's unwise to become dependent on herbal laxatives. There is no substitute for an excellent fibrous diet to cleanse the bowels as well as bring down bad cholesterol naturally.

DON'T FORGET THE SKIN

The skin, as we saw in chapter 1, is the largest organ and one of our best eliminative organs of our body. Skin cleansing is therefore a vital part of the detoxification process, particularly when it comes to the heavy metals (aluminum and mercury) that are eliminated through the skin's pores when we sweat. Consistent exercise, steam rooms, and sauna baths are excellent ways to remove toxins from the skin and maximize your health.

Basic skin care is a daily matter, beginning with using natural soaps when you bathe. Skin care products made from chemicals may be cheaper, but remember that those chemicals *will* be absorbed into the bloodstream. Though the amount may be small, it is the cumulative effect of the chemicals that damages your health over the long run. If your body has a toxicity problem, you will notice the difference when you move to natural products on your body. Especially stay away from sodium laurel sulfate—a known carcinogen.

Dry skin brushing is easy to do and helps in removing the outer dead skin layers and keeps the pores open. You will need to buy a natural bristle brush or bath mitt and expect to spend five minutes for brushing your skin. Use light pressure and a circular motion, then shower and moisturize your skin. When detoxifying, the cellular turnover on the skin speeds up, and thus the dead cells coming off will be greater!

Another good technique for cleansing the skin is to towel off roughly until the skin gets slightly red. It will only take you a few minutes more than usual.

Food grade hydrogen peroxide baths are excellent for energy and detoxifying. Epsom salts baths are also very good. For each bath you will need between 8-16 ounces of Epsom salts and 3 ounces of sea salt. Run comfortable warm water and add the salts and dissolve them. Soak for 10-20 minutes and then scrub the skin gently with soap on a natural fiber. Within a few minutes the water will turn murky. The darkness to the water is because of heavy metals coming out of the skin. Get out of the bath carefully, as you may feel light-headed. Then wrap yourself in several towels (you may sweat heavily afterward) and go to bed. Make sure you have water at your bedside because you will be thirsty. Do this once a week during a detoxification program, but once a month is sufficient normally.

Good skin care also requires good nutrition and an abundance of water. Since your skin is mainly fat, you need high-quality fats and oils from natural sources to keep your skin healthy. Olive oil is an excellent source as well as evening primrose and Vitamin E, and combinations of essential fatty acids.

"Friendly" Bacteria

A key to improving our digestive functions, the immune system, and overall health is the constant restoration of healthy intestinal flora ("friendly" bacteria). It is such an important part of your detoxification process that I devoted an entire chapter to it in *"Candida Albicans"* (chapter 5). I go into detail on the essential role of the normal flora of our gastrointestinal track to defend our body from the pathogenic species of bacteria and to perform many vital functions, one of which is the detoxification of toxic chemicals. When our normal flora are present, they secrete mediators in which the pathogenic forms cannot grow.

However, antibiotics kill off the good bacteria as well as the bad and allow the bad to repopulate and develop antibiotic resistance. Natural forms of antibiotics are better, since they do not kill off the good bacteria with the bad and do not allow drug resistance to take place. Fresh, raw garlic, for example, has strong antimicrobial power and is more effective against pathogens than most antibiotics today. Herbal antiseptics and antibacterial tonics are far better and less dangerous to our health than antibiotics.

Replacing our natural flora is a good step for preventing disease and keeping our bowels healthy. Check out the "Treatment for *Candida Albicans*" on page 89 to learn about restoring the health of your flora.

Herbal Power

Detoxification diets are the primary means to cleansing

your system, and herbs have been used medicinally for centuries to supplement the cleansing of the blood and tissues or strengthening the function of specific organs. Many herbs have been proven as powerful neutraceutical agents that can support or even cause detoxification. There are hundreds of possible medicinal herbs, and they also provide vitamins, minerals, and enzymes for excellent nutrition. I have a large section on herbs in the "Nature's Prescriptions for Feeling Great" (chapter 11) that will help direct you in this area. It includes a chart showing herbal alternatives to drugs, essential medicinal herbs, and specific concerns about herbs.

Herbs can be combined together to fortify those specific herbs that aid specific organs. These are found commonly in organic food stores. But it is possible for herbs to interact negatively with one another. If you suspect a bad interaction, consult your physician or pharmacist.

Herbs may be used as teas, salves, tinctures, poultices, capsules, tablets, and concentrated extracts. Always follow the manufacturer's advice regarding the dose. Herbal teas are an easy way to start to enhance your health throughout the day. They are a delicious substitute to break the coffee habit and a potent source of health modulators.

Many people utilize an herbal cleanse. For example, first thing in the morning they may drink a glass of steam-distilled water with a teaspoon of blackstrap molasses and a teaspoon of apple cider vinegar added. During the morning they drink a glass of water with psyllium husk powder, which they follow with a second glass of water. During their meals they take digestive enzymes. Between meals they may take liver herbs and drink herbal teas that specifically help support the liver.

THE FIGHT AGAINST FREE RADICALS

In the process of metabolism or oxidation, our body cells produce molecules called free radicals. They are unstable molecules that attempt to steal electrons from any available source, such as our body tissues. Antioxidants, such as beta-carotene, Vitamins A, E, and especially C, and selenium, work to neutralize these unstable chemicals and protect us from them. Vitamin C is very essential to any detoxification programs because the body uses it for energy to process and eliminate these toxic wastes. The more antioxidants we get in our diets, the more we are able to stop these damaging effects. The main source of antioxidants is fruits, vegetables, nuts, grains, and cold-pressed plant oils.

Antioxidants are essential for detoxification because they help cells neutralize free radicals that can cause mutations and cellular damage. This damage is partly responsible for a wide range of illnesses, including all the degenerative diseases such as arthritis, cardiovascular disease, Alzheimer's, and cancer. Any shortage of antioxidants can become catastrophic to one's health. When our antioxidants are low, energy is not available and detoxification cannot take place in a normal fashion. Therefore, toxins accumulate or are stored until they can be processed.

Other excellent sources of antioxidants are found in bioflavonoids, grape seed extract, ginseng, garlic, molybdenum,

DHEA, wheat and barley grass, Echinacea, manganese, carotenoids, Ginkgo Biloba, melatonin, L-Cysteine, acetyl-l-carnite, CoQ10, milk thistle, and B-vitamins.

YOU ARE WHAT YOU ABSORB

Enzymes have a major impact on your health and detoxification. They help digest and absorb proteins, carbohydrates or starches, lipids or fats. Absorption is absolutely crucial to your health. They also clean up dead tissues, enhance your own enzyme capacity, and help the bowels in cleansing, because they liquefy the bowel content and make for a quicker passage. The quicker the toxins are out of your system, the better your health is, and the better you feel!

While vitamins and minerals get significant attention, don't minimize the role of enzymes. Vitamins and minerals are used to activate enzymes, but enzymes do the hard work of detoxifying toxins and supporting the metabolism of the body.

The best source of enzymes is fresh raw fruits and vegetables, which can be supplemented with multidigestive enzymes. Unfortunately, enzymes are destroyed by processing and cooking. If you eat a high proportion of processed foods, you lose out on these vital ingredients. By eating a wide range of foods, as close to their raw state as possible, you can enjoy all these benefits.

The liver is the source of most detoxification enzymes, which it either makes or stores. To aid the liver in removing and eliminating wastes and toxins, enzymes are best taken with meals. This way they aid in digestion.

MERCURY TOXICITY

While it is beyond the scope of this book to cover the dangers of mercury toxicity related to dental fillings, the fact is that mercury comprises about 50 percent of the most common filling in the world called silver-mercury amalgam. This amalgam also contains copper, tin, silver, and zinc. There are many factors that can increase the release of mercury emissions into your system, but the fact that mercury is released at all is scary. Many experts feel that the amount of mercury released is adequate to contribute significantly to disease processes.

Where does all the mercury go? Into your body. Absorption of mercury occurs the fastest from the area under your tongue and the insides of your cheeks. Being in such close proximity to the fillings, the efficiency of absorption is great. From these tissues, the mercury can destroy adjacent tissues or travel to the lymphatic drainage system and directly into the bloodstream. From the bloodstream, mercury can travel to any cell in the body, where it can either disable or destroy the tissues. Mercury can also travel directly from the fillings into the lungs, where it then enters into the bloodstream, and every cell in the body becomes a potential target.

The ability of mercury to travel throughout the body and its accompanying destruction are what define mercury toxicity. It may favor nerve tissue for a destruction target, but the kidney is high up on its hit list. After these two areas, it can wreak havoc in any tissue that gets in its way.

It can alter almost anything in the body; therefore, mercury should not be allowed to enter for any reason.

This is especially problematic if someone has a tooth or teeth that have leached a significant amount of mercury into the body. Detoxification will not help to any great extent until the mercury is taken out. Many of the doctors listed in the back of this book will not even do chelation or treat new patients until the mercury is eliminated or the entire tooth is removed.

THE HEALING CRISIS

In the fasting chapter, I address this more fully because of the intensity of fasting's detoxification process. Nevertheless, even during milder detoxification programs, it is possible for your body to detoxify too rapidly and have toxins released faster than the body can eliminate them. When this occurs, you may suffer from headaches, nausea, vomiting, depression, and even old aches and pains you forgot you had! This is a good thing! It means your body is working. If this occurs, back off the program and proceed at a slower pace. Forcing a detoxification process too quickly can have negative results.

According to naturopathic theory, any symptoms of the disease that have previously been experienced may also be experienced transiently during detoxification, and I have seen this occur quite often. However, sometimes it's difficult to know what is going on inside. Should you treat the problems that come up or simply watch them? Since my basic approach is to allow the body to heal itself and support the natural healing process whenever possible, that is what I try to do unless it becomes intolerable.

For many of us, especially the new or inexperienced, it is wise to begin any special program, diet, or lifestyle changes with a few days at home or possibly over a weekend. In time, experience will tell you what is best. Most of us can maintain a regular work schedule during a cleanse or detoxification program (you'll probably feel great), but it may be easier to begin a program on a Friday, as the first few days are usually the hardest.

FASTING

FASTING IS A PERIOD OF RE-STRICTED FOOD INTAKE THAT DETOXIFIES THE BODY, GIVING THE ORGANS A REST AND BRING-ING NATURAL HEALING BY CLEANSING THE BODY. But fasting is not only excellent for the body, it is also breath to the spirit as well. God says in Isaiah 58 that He has a chosen fast that is redemptive for every area of your life. Your spirit, mind, and body are included so that no disease will come upon you! Fasting facilitates this divine freedom. "Then your light will break forth like the dawn, and your healing will quickly appear." Your fast can be a time to be restored to a right relationship with Him! He will go before you as your righteousness, and His glory will be your guardian.

What a marvelous incentive to begin a fast! Blessings to all who choose to make this exciting healing journey! May your health spring forth speedily. God will be with you!

Fasting has been practiced for centuries among many societies, particularly for religious purposes. Among the Jews, the Day of Atonement was the most prominent occasion for a public fast (Leviticus 16:29-31; 23:27-36; Numbers 29:7). The Old Testament also refers to many special fasts, both public and individual (Judges 20:26; 1 Samuel 14:24; 31:13; 2 Samuel 1:12; 12:16-23; 1 Kings 21:27; 2 Chronicles 20:3). Jesus Christ was led by the Spirit to a forty day and night fast in the desert, which was followed by a time of intense temptation (Matthew 4:1-11). He gave His followers instructions for how He wanted them to fast (Matthew 6:16-18), and there is clear evidence of fasting in the early church (Acts 13:2-3; 14:23).

WHAT ARE THE BENEFITS?

I have seen in my fasting and *Candida* clinic that fasting is both a primary means of detoxifying the body, shedding unwanted pounds, and a wonderful aid to spiritual renewal. While our emphasis for purposes of feeling great focuses on the cleansing of the body and weight loss, keep in mind that the health of your spiritual life is intrinsic to your overall health. There is no substitute for experiencing on a daily basis the fullness of joy from being in a right relationship with God.

Fasting has been proven to be the most effective means of getting the body into a natural healing process. It is also an instrument to literally reset the body's odometer and help reverse the aging process. Disease and aging begin when the normal process of cell regeneration and rebuilding slows down. This slowdown is caused by the accumulation of waste products in the tissues, which interferes with the nourishment and oxygenation of cells. This may happen at any age, and when it occurs, the cells' resistance to disease diminishes and various ills start to appear. Given the fact that at any given moment one-fourth of all our cells are dead and in replacement, it is of vital importance that the dying cells are decomposed and eliminated from the system as efficiently as possible. Quick and effective elimination of dead cells stimulates the building and growth of new cells.

Hippocrates (c. 460-377 B.C.), the Greek physician often called "the father of medicine," spoke of this well over two thousand years ago. He said, "Food should be our medicine, and medicine should be our food, but to eat when you are sick is to feed your illness." Such ancient advice contains true wisdom. When you stop eating, your organs rest, and all the energy in your body is directed to healing.

By ridding the body of toxicity, you will find yourself more alert and energetic, requiring less sleep, and you will experience a keener sense of awareness to those around you as well as to your own spirit and the Holy Spirit. In simple words, you will find yourself being led by your spirit and not by your appetite.

In Germany, Dr. Otto Buchinger Jr., who is an authority on fasting, has supervised over 90,000 successful fasting and detox programs and has used these methods to treat virtually every disease—rheumatic conditions, digestive disorders, skin conditions, cardiovascular disorders, and more. Diminished hormone levels can be restored simply by cleansing the body.

We now know that by fasting only three days a month, you can increase your life-span by five to seven years. An interesting study was conducted in Europe with centenarians (those living to be over one hundred years of age). The study showed that there was only one common link among this age group—they all ate less than the average person, and they fasted often! Cornell University studies have shown that by keeping animals from overeating and implementing systematic fasting, their lives can be increased up to 50 percent.

Another study, called "The Hunger Treatment," was conducted in Russia in 1986 at a hospital for the mentally ill. The study lasted for sixty days and involved eight hundred schizophrenics who were made to partake in a juice fast. After only 25-30 days of cleansing, 64 percent of the patients improved mentally, which led to the assessment that two-thirds of the patients diagnosed with mental problems were actually in such a state of toxicity that the brain could not function properly. Since that study we know that many misdiagnosed mental illnesses can be attributed to heavy metal poisoning as well as a lack of nutrients. By giving the patient the right nutrients, balance can occur and health be restored.

HOW FASTING WORKS

Fasting means to not eat, but it doesn't mean you should restrict yourself to water only. In fact, juice fasting has proven to be the most effective way to restore your health back to the way God intended.

During a prolonged fast (after the first three days), your body will live on its own substance. When it is deprived of needed nutrition, particularly of proteins and fats, it will burn and digest its own tissues by the process of *autolysis,* or self-digestion. But your body will not do this indiscriminately! Through the divine wisdom of our Great Creator, your body will first decompose and burn those cells and tissues that are diseased, damaged, aged, or dead. In the fasting process, your body feeds itself on the most impure and inferior materials, such as dead cells and morbid accumulations—tumors, abscesses, fat deposits, etc. Dr. Buchinger says, "Fasting is a refuse disposal, a burning of rubbish." The essential body tissues and vital organs, the glands, the nervous system, and the brain are not damaged or digested in a fast.

In general, three- to ten-day fasts are recommended for health and longevity. The body needs three to five days of fasting to actually begin the autolysis process whereby the body attacks inferior matter in the body and begins the healing process. A five-day fast essentially clears debris before disease gets started. A ten-day fast works to attack disease that has already begun and often eliminates problems from the body before the symptoms arise. During the fast, the function of the eliminative organs—liver, kidneys, lungs, and the skin—is greatly increased, and accumulated toxins and waste are quickly expelled. During the fast, toxins in the urine can be ten times higher than normal.

HOW TO FAST

If you have never fasted before, it is best to start with several one-day fasts before moving on to a three-day fast. Do these once a week until you feel comfortable moving on.

Then have a three-day fast once a month. As a preparation for it, reduce the amount of food and eat only whole raw organic foods two to three days before you begin your fast. I recommend beginning the fast on a Friday evening and extending it through Monday evening. Most people are at home on weekends and can easily do their juicing and cleansing with few interruptions. For many people the second day feels the worst, so it's best to have that on a day of rest. Think of it as a time to give your body a rest, to let it retune itself, and to aid in its healing process.

Start each day of your fast with room temperature steam-distilled water. Every day you should be drinking half of your body weight in ounces of water. For example, if you weigh 150 pounds, drink 75 ounces of water each day. Health science consensus currently believes that steam-distilled water is the best for fasting as well as daily use. Steam-distilled water is the only water that actually goes in and pulls out toxins from the organs. It literally pulls out the mire that gets caught in the follicles of the colon and breeds disease. You will also find that steam-distilled water helps curb your appetite, unlike drinks or juice that causes your body to want more.

The best juices are the ones you juice yourself. Fresh organic veggies are in supply at your local health food store as well as grocery stores. Stock up on the freshest you can find. During a fast, my favorite juice is a carrot, beet, and ginger combination. Feel free to use a variety of veggies and fruits. Fresh lemon, cabbage, beet, carrot, grape (including the seeds), apple (skin and seeds), green combos made from leafy greens such as spinach, kale, turnips, etc.—these are all excellent detoxifiers.

Raw cabbage juice is known to aid in the recovery from ulcers, cancer, and all colon problems. However, it must be fresh, not stored. Cabbage loses its Vitamin U content after sitting for only a short time.

Another excellent juice blend is three carrots, two stalks of celery, one turnip, two beets, a half head of cabbage, a quarter bunch of parsley, and a clove of garlic. This could be one of the best juices on our planet for the restoration of the body from many ailments.

Another favorite juice preparation is Stanley Borroughs's "Master Cleanser." In a gallon of steam-distilled water, mix the juice of five fresh lemons and a half cup of grade B maple syrup. Add one or more tablespoons of hot cayenne pepper (at least 90,000 heat units) to your taste tolerance. This is especially good for alkalinizing the body and raising body temperature to help resolve infection and flu-type illnesses.

Pure vegetable broths with no seasonings added are also good. To prepare these, gently boil vegetables, including lots of onions and garlic, for 30 minutes. Do not eat the stew, but strain the broth and drink the juice two or three times a day.

The juices, broths, and water will keep you adequately full as well as provide you with more nutrients than most people normally get from their diets. If you must eat something, have a slice of watermelon. Organic grapes with seeds are also good, especially Concord grapes, which have a powerful antioxidant effect. Alternatively, fresh applesauce made with the skins on and the seeds intact, processed in a blender or food processor, is satisfying and won't significantly disrupt your fast.

A great way to top off your day, whether fasting or not, is to have a half cup of oat bran with a non-dairy milk (soy, almond, or rice). This helps to cleanse the colon by adding fiber and has been shown to cut the risk of cancer by 30 percent! I have found that eating oat bran before going to bed suits my body well and seems to aid in a peaceful night's rest.

Green drinks can also be an added bonus to any fast. We have created one called *Creation's Bounty*, which is a whole raw organic food with all the nutrients your body needs. There may also be other green drinks to choose from at your local health food store.

DAILY SUGGESTED PROTOCOL FOR YOUR FAST

- Start with 4-8 ounces of *Clustered Water*™. This will help to clean the lymphatic system.
- Fifteen minutes later take 1-2 ounces of *Body Oxygen*™.
- Thirty to forty minutes later have a green drink.
- Prepare your favorite fresh juice combination, which you can alternate with Stanley Burroughs's lemonade drink. If you don't have a juicer, use the best organic juice from your grocery store.

- Prepare fresh vegetables broth to sip in between juices and/or green smoothies.
- Remember to drink as much steam-distilled water as possible.
- A good liquid mineral supplement will aid in rapid healing.
- If you must eat, remember—grapes, watermelon, or fresh applesauce.
- Rest whenever you feel weak during a fast. Deep-breathing exercises and frequent showers are helpful.

FASTING DON'TS

- Don't fast on water alone!
- Don't chew gum or mints. This starts the digestive juices flowing and is harmful to the system. When your stomach releases hydrochloric acid in the gut, but nothing ever gets down there, is it a surprise that you have a stomachache?
- Don't drink orange or tomato juice on a fast. They are too acidic.
- Don't ever eat junk foods, especially before the fast. The last food you eat will be the next food you crave. If you eat junk food, you'll want more of it. If you eat veggies, you'll want something healthy. Our bodies are designed by God to want healthy food, but when we eat the wrong things, we deaden our senses to what is good. Did you ever notice when you eat a fast-food burger you feel full for about 30 minutes, and then suddenly you're hungry again! This is because your body is so desperate for nutrition it is still trying to get you to

eat something it can actually benefit from instead of dead, unbeneficial calories?

EXTENDED FASTS

There are fasts that last up to 100 days. Twenty-, thirty-, and forty-day fasts are common to individuals with extraordinary needs. These fasts must be scientifically supervised, though, and not just undertaken at will. Proper liquid nutrition must be ingested, and additional supplementation may be required. Your program must be tailor-made for you and your personal makeup. For individuals with these needs, such as extreme obesity, disease, etc., I recommend that you contact a specialist in the back of this book or call my office at 817-236-8557.

WHILE YOU FAST

When going on a juice fast of three days or longer, some experts advise taking an herbal laxative on the first day of the fast and every two or three days during a longer fast. I prefer and personally recommend enemas during a fast as an absolute must. Enemas assist the body in its detoxifying effort by cleansing out all the toxic waste from the alimentary canal. A healthy, normal adult is carrying around 7-14 pounds of waste (that's the weight of a new-born baby!). Think of what an immune-compromised or overweight person may have stored up. People continually ask me why they are still having large bowel movements after several days of not eating. The answer is simple—most people have years of backup to clean out.

Enemas should be taken at least once, preferably twice, a day during your fast—one after rising in the morning and the other before going to bed. One pint to one quart of lukewarm distilled water is sufficient. Enema bags are available in any drugstore. One word of medical caution—enemas tend to delete the potassium level, therefore care must be taken for proper supplementation.

An excellent way to stimulate the liver to detoxify itself during a fast is with coffee enemas. This we refer to as a "Liver Cleanse." You'll find information regarding this in the Question and Answer section.

Although naturopaths have used both enemas and colonic irrigation for many years in their detoxification methods, its use is not without controversy. Fiber supplements are now available that can be taken by mouth and achieve similar purposes.

MAINTENANCE AFTER A FAST

Fasting brings the body back to doing what it is designed to do, which is for you to accomplish the will of God without the hindrances of fatigue, obesity, and illness. Most people, following initial withdrawal from chemical dependencies (including caffeine and sugar), dramatically see and feel a difference in their health status by day three of a good fast. People commonly feel lighter and more energized and notice improvements in complexion and eye color. These changes indicate you are on your way back to optimal health.

Always break the fast gently. Whole raw organic foods may be used. Nothing heavy or chemical laden should be eaten, such as processed foods. For powerful aid in rebuilding the immune system before and after the fast, drink Pau d'arco and Echinacea tea mixed with one-third unsweetened cranberry juice four times a day.

Lightly steamed vegetables in their broth with whole grain brown rice can be added slowly and used as part of a maintenance diet.

DEALING WITH THE HEALING CRISIS

When you alter your diet, especially during a fast, changes occur that are often misunderstood. Far too often I have seen individuals who were properly detoxing, cleansing, and healing quit just before the finish line. This is simply due to misunderstanding the way the body was designed by God to heal itself. The following will hopefully give you clarity as to what to expect when you are in the eliminative process that brings healing. Remember, the Word says, "At the proper time we will reap a harvest if we do not give up" (Galatians 6:9).

Dr. Bernard Jensen has defined a healing crisis as "an acute reaction resulting from the ascendance of the natural healing forces over disease conditions. Its tendency is toward recovery, and it is, therefore, in conformity with the natural reconstruction principle put innately in us by God." It is the direct result of an industrious effort of every organ in the body to eliminate waste products and set the stage for regeneration. Through this constructive process toward health, old tissues are replaced with new.

In a healing crisis there is usually a fever, which shows

that the body is fighting to burn out residues of old viruses, bacteria, and disease in general. Symptoms of the healing crisis may at first be identical to the disease it is meant to heal. But the real distinction is elimination. Elimination is usually significantly increased, due to the fact that all the eliminative organs are doing their part to rid the body of harmful toxins and buildup. This is just the opposite in a diseased state, when the body is usually either constipated or very irregular, leaving the body in an unsatisfactory condition and compounding the trouble. When elimination occurs, you know that the body is in a purifying and cleansing process.

In time the new tissue becomes strong enough to take its place in the various activities of the body. The old tissue is expelled through various means—phlegm, mucous, sweat, bowels, etc. As the process of building up new cellular structure has been accomplished, the real healing is taking place.

According to Dr. Jensen, there are three stages to the healing crisis:

- Eliminative—the body ridding itself of debris.
- Transitional—new tissue is maturing.
- Building—the body is then going into homeostasis, a state of health, the way God intended us to live.

A healing crisis usually lasts about three days. During that time, various aches, pains, and symptoms of ailments from long ago seem to rear their ugly head. Some people only experience a slight headache, while others may feel as if they are on their last leg. All of this is dependent upon the degree of cleansing the body needs to accomplish. If the crisis is bearable, work through it, as the rewards are well worth it. If it is unbearable, back off slightly, then try again later. The body will order each step of the crisis from the inside out and from the head down, which is why it usually starts with a headache.

Please keep in mind that the majority of physical problems the average American is facing is brought on by a poor diet, lack of exercise, and a fast-pace stressful lifestyle. Fasting and detoxing assist in ridding the body of the lifestyle buildups that eventually develop into chronic diseases. One healing crisis may not be enough for complete restoration. You may require a number of cycles of healing crises. Think of it as peeling the layers off an onion.

Keep in mind that the crisis is necessary in order for true healing to take place. You must get rid of the old to bring in the new. Just think of the whole body getting into action to correct ailing organs, joints, and various conditions in the body. True healing can never occur without a real cleansing of the eliminative organs.

After the healing crisis has occurred, strength, energy, and health begin to build. After a cleanse, a healthy diet, proper amounts of oxygen, good water and lots of it, along with a moderate exercise program, you will be giving your body what it needs to stay on track.

As always, you may want to consult your physician regarding any concerns you have about symptoms during what you perceive to be a healing crisis. It is easy to mistake serious medical symptoms for minor symptoms. And always check with your physician before beginning any new cleansing or exercise program.

RESTORE YOUR SYSTEM TO GOD'S PLAN

*Daniel then said to the guard
whom the chief official had appointed over
Daniel, Hananiah, Mishael and Azariah, "Please
test your servants for ten days: Give us nothing
but vegetables to eat and water to drink.
Then compare our appearance with that
of the young men who eat the royal food, and treat
your servants in accordance with what you see."
So he agreed to this and tested them for ten days.
At the end of the ten days they looked healthier
and better nourished than any of the young men who
ate the royal food. So the guard took away their
choice food and the wine they were to drink
and gave them vegetables instead.*

DANIEL 1:11-16

REDUCING YOUR TEMPLE THROUGH WEIGHT LOSS

- **YOU ARE CHOSEN BY GOD** FOR SUCH A TIME AS THIS!
- You have the call of God on your life!
- You have a destiny to fulfill!
- You are on this earth at the right time!
- These are the last days!

You're probably thinking this is a very strange introduction for a weight-loss plan. Quite the contrary! The most important reason you should ever want to lose weight is to empower you so that you can fulfill God's will for your life. The Bible tells us that the gifts and callings of God are irrevocable or without repentance (Romans 11:29). However, we are the ones who should repent for allowing anything in our lives to hold us back from performing God's will in the earth today.

God will never take back His plan for your life. He is simply waiting for you to lay aside every weight that so easily hinders and entangles you (Hebrews 12:1). He desires that you be "forgetting what is behind and straining toward what is ahead . . . press on toward the goal to win the prize for which God has called [you] heavenward in Christ Jesus" (Philippians 3:13-14). Whatever your calling in life, it is a high calling. You are valuable in the eyes of God. I encourage you to read this chapter with an open mind, a tender heart, and an ear to hear our God speak to you about the relationship of your health, your weight, and His plan for your life. As a part of the "Body of Christ," make sure that your part of the Body is healthy.

Please pray this prayer with me: "Father, I want to be used by You. I desire to be a vessel You can work through. Please show me how I can take better care of this beautiful temple You have given me. Help me to fulfill the blueprint You have designed for me and only me—the one no one else can fill. Please show me who I am in You and how I can be a blessing to the Kingdom of God. In Jesus' name, amen!"

I pray many blessings upon you, the chief of which is that you prosper and be in health. I am in agreement with your desire for a whole and healthy body.

WISDOM

In Proverbs, it says that the Lord gives wisdom and from His mouth come knowledge and understanding (Proverbs 2:6). We all need wisdom in our daily lives, but many times we do not think of asking for wisdom in small things. There is nothing too small to bring before God the Father. In the Kingdom of God, there is no such thing as a small prayer. Any prayer asked in faith is pleasing to God. Your prayer may be, "Lord, what do you want me to eat today?" or, "Lord, what is Your will for my life?" The Bible says that He is moved with the feelings of our weaknesses (Hebrews 4:15). And it also says to cast all your cares on Him, because He cares for you (Philippians 4:6). In other words, if it concerns you, it concerns Him.

So for your first weight-loss assignment, pray and ask the Lord to give you His wisdom. Ask Him to reveal the changes that you need to make to achieve your desired goal. If you need some help knowing what to pray, simply pray this: "Heavenly Father, You tell me in Your Word that I am to get wisdom, so, Lord, I am asking for Your wisdom in my life. Father, I ask You to reveal the changes I need to make in order to achieve my weight-loss goals. Lord, help me to listen to You and follow Your leading in this area of my life. I want a strong, healthy body, and I am tired of fighting a weight problem. I cast the care of it on you right now. Thank you for hearing my prayer and answering it. In Jesus' mighty name, amen."

THE BIG PROBLEM AND THE GOAL

An estimated 300,000 Americans die prematurely each year of disease caused by being very overweight. Americans eat 300-400 percent more fat than they should, and 800 percent more than they need! Approximately one-quarter to one-third of adults in the United States are classified as overweight, depending on the BMI (body mass index, weight/height) cut point used. The prevalence of over-weight people has increased during the last two decades.

A serious health problem exists all around us. We see one group of people who do not need to lose weight but are trying anyway. We also see thousands of people who do need to lose weight yet are not succeeding. The percentage of Americans whose health and longevity are jeopardized by too much weight is increasing, and thus our focus is with this group. It is associated with elevated cholesterol levels, elevated blood pressure, and noninsulin-dependent diabetes mellitus. Excessive weight also increases the risk for coronary heart disease, gallbladder disease, gout, some types of cancer, and has been implicated in the development of osteoarthritis of the weight-bearing joints.

The following guidelines are for general use. Although there is agreement among government and scientific groups about the general range of BMI that constitutes a healthy weight, agreement on an exact range has not been established. The range varies according to age and gender. For example, bone structure and body type will certainly play key roles in determining what your ideal weight should be, so factor those in.

Women. Typically, we start with 100 pounds for the first five feet and then add 5 pounds for every inch after that to calculate a female's weight. For example, a five-foot-six-inch woman should weigh in the neighborhood of 130 pounds. A five-foot-one-inch woman should weigh around 105 pounds.

Men. The guideline begins the same; however, instead of 5 pounds for every inch over five feet, add 7 to 10 pounds. For example, a six-foot-one-inch man should weigh anywhere from 190 pounds to 220 pounds, depending on bone structure and body type. A five-foot-eight-inch man with a small frame may feel quite comfortable at 150 pounds.

I tell people to go by how they feel. Ladies, do you feel healthier when you wear a size 10 or a size 14? Men, do you feel stronger when you have a 34-inch waistline or more comfortable when you're between a 38-inch and a 40-inch waist? Your body will speak to you. Just listen. It is giving you signals, such as fatigue, poor digestion, high blood pressure, high cholesterol, constipation, joint pain, and the list goes on. Also, remember that muscle weighs three times more than fat, so if you start working out you may measure smaller but weigh more!

Weight-loss benefits are numerous. Here are a few of the major ones if drop your body weight by *just 10 percent:*

- A healthier heart. You can lower your cholesterol and reduce your blood pressure through weight loss. High cholesterol and elevated blood pressure are two major risk factors for heart disease.
- Lower risk of Type 2 Diabetes. Overweight people are at an increased risk for Type 2 Diabetes, which occurs when your body can't make enough, or properly use, insulin, a hormone that helps convert food to usable energy. Weight loss improves your body's ability to use the insulin it makes, possibly preventing the onset of the disease.
- More energy. Expect to feel better, full of vigor and vitality.
- New self-confidence. Success in weight loss builds your self-confidence and increases your motivation to keep going. When you look better and feel better, you're only going to want to improve your overall health as well as continue to shed any extra pounds that need to go.
- People who are slightly underweight live longer.
- Age slower.

WHAT NEXT?

Now that you have prayed for God to give you wisdom and determined what your ideal weight should be, it's time for goal setting.

Remember, you didn't get where you are overnight, and you won't get back to where you want to be overnight either—not safely anyway. Most people have let their bodies go for years, and then when they decide they're ready to lose weight, they want it to happen instantly. But it just doesn't work that way. Losing 50 pounds in a month is not healthy, no matter how great it sounds. We need to set realistic goals to accomplish permanent weight-loss results.

Let me explain the process of weight loss so that you won't be discouraged along the way to a thinner and healthier you. Initially, you will lose weight quickly as your body burns glucose. Then, as your body begins to lose fat, the weight will come off slower, but that weight loss will be more of a permanent weight loss—not just a few quick pounds of glucose and water.

We want the extra pounds to come off for good, and to do that, we need to do it the right way and get to the root of the problem. No more of this human yo-yo with weight loss again: up some months, and down for others. The human yo-yo routine is never healthy, and it is very defeating to the mind and spirit. So set your goals in accordance with God's plan for your life and for your body type. A good goal to start with would be 15-20 pounds the first month and then 10-15 pounds the following months, depending, of course, upon how much you need to lose.

LET'S GET STARTED ✍

One of the worst disappointments in the world is to set a goal, get all psyched up about it, start on a program, and then crash and burn soon after beginning. We've all done it! Then, that evil spirit of defeat comes knocking at your door with plenty of guilt and condemnation. Here's some really good advice—don't answer! Jesus, the Son of God, is the only person who did not fail His mission. If you fail, it just means you're human. Determine right now that you will keep trying until you succeed.

I'm going to let you in on a little secret to help you get started on the right foot—there could be critters living on the inside of that human body of yours that are sabotaging your weight-loss efforts! Yes, I mean parasites, and most likely *Candida Albicans*. We all have these yeast-like anaerobic bacteria. It's just to what extent that makes the difference.

You may think you simply have no will power, but it might just be those critters telling your brain you need a snack. That's what *Candida* does. They crave sugars and yeast products such as breads. These sugary, high-carbohydrate foods feed the *Candida*, and when you ingest sugar, they thrive and the cravings get stronger and stronger. It becomes a vicious cycle, while all along you think it's you!

I encourage you, before you begin to "Reduce Your Temple," to read chapter 5 on *Candida* and take the Self-Analysis Test. Determine if you should start with a *Candida* cleanse, which will assist you in losing weight, because the sugar and high carbohydrate cravings will be stifled before you get started.

COMPLETING THE WORK

After completing the *Candida* cleanse, you should have rid your body of most of those little critters that make you crave the very foods you shouldn't eat. I say most, because *Candida* will hide in the body, and if you go back to a diet heavy in sugars, starches, and breads, it will start its growth pattern all over again and sabotage your goal at weight loss.

Now it's time to move forward with a good fasting program that will quickly rid your body of toxins. Besides the immense value of detoxing the body, fasting will also shrink your stomach, which will jump-start your weight-loss program naturally. In my chapter on fasting, I go into great detail on how to have a successful fast for three or more days.

If fasting sounds scary to you, be assured that the fasting program I have designed provides all the nutrients you should be getting during this time. Fasting is good for you, and you can do it!

Now, make a fist, then examine the size of it. Did you know that this is the size of your very own empty stomach? Now, open your hand flat—that is the size your stomach should be when you are full. Compare that to your average plate of food. Interesting, huh?

TIME TO EXERCISE!

Okay, we're off to a good start! Now that you have a clean temple, you can start the remodeling process. It's time to *exercise!* There is no way around it. There is no magic pill that will keep the weight off. You just gotta do it!

When you were fasting, your body was burning stored glucose, and you were probably going to the bathroom a lot. When glucose is not burned up every day, it is stored in the body along with water. When you fast, the glucose is used by the mitochondria (think of them as tiny power plants) in the cells, causing you to lose weight as well as to urinate often. This is often referred to as the loss of "water weight," which usually happens rather quickly and is very encouraging. It will be the fastest weight you lose during your program.

But the next step is what really counts. Burning fat! After the excess glucose is utilized, then the body will start to burn fat, which burns at a much slower rate than glucose. So although the scale moves down much slower, don't be discouraged. Good work is being accomplished!

Exercise is key in weight loss because when you exercise, you burn calories. And when you burn calories, the body must compensate for the extra energy being used, so the mitochondria inside your cells divide. Since the mitochondria act as our power plants, burning fuel, they divide as you exercise, burning twice as much. Nothing else will do that. Realize that by exercising, the body will compensate by burning more fat. It's that simple.

So are you psyched to exercise? Chapter 4 provides you with a successful program to help you get started, no matter how badly you are out of shape. I've watched people who could barely lift 5 pounds move up to 30 pounds in just a few short weeks. You can do it! You must do it!

Here's the good news. After those first few days of exercise, you will have more energy, you will sleep better, your body will start looking good, your stamina will increase, and best of all, you will be burning more fat! You will also have a better mental attitude, and your stress level will dramatically decrease. All of which translates into weight loss!

Determine today to make time for exercise. Make it a part of your daily routine, and before long, you'll wonder how you ever lived without it! You'll actually start enjoying exercise because you'll feel so good and look great, too!

WHAT TO EAT

After completing the *Candida* cleanse, going on a minimum of a three-day fast, and beginning an exercise program, you need to know what you can take in on a daily basis. It's not the time to splurge because you've lost 10 pounds. It's the time to dig in and complete your course. So here are some guidelines to help you finish the race.

The following is a step-by-step program to reduce your temple. With the emphasis on making the noon meal your biggest meal of the day, it may require that you rearrange your schedule a bit to prepare your food ahead of time. Don't be discouraged, though. Think of it as though you're simply packing a lunch box before you leave home!

- When you first awake, drink 6-8 ounces of *Clustered Water™*.
- Within 10-15 minutes take two ounces of *Body Oxygen™*.

- Wait at least 15-20 minutes before taking in anything else.
- In a blender, mix one cup of yogurt without added sugar, one freckled banana, 6 ounces of apple juice, soy or rice milk, one heaping scoop of *Creation's Bounty*, and fill the balance with a few ice cubes and distilled water. Drink as much as you like, then continue to drink it throughout the morning. Feel free to substitute any other fresh fruit that blends well, such as strawberries or peaches without added sugar. You can use different juices. Just be sure nothing is added, such as sugar, Aspartame™, Sweet & Low™, chemicals, etc. These synthetic sweeteners are now being linked to Type 2 Diabetes, also known as Syndrome X.
- While you have the shake on your stomach, you may want to try an ephedra-free energy supplement with plenty of B vitamins included.
- Every day drink half your body weight in ounces of water. Feel free to drink more if you'd like.
- Midmorning, have a fresh piece of fruit, preferably a type of melon in season.
- Approximately 15 minutes before you are planning to eat lunch, such as when you begin the meal preparation, eat five almonds. This will send a signal to the brain to tell you that you are full.
- For lunch, have a piece of broiled or baked fish, or tuna without the mayo (you can substitute plain yogurt in tuna salad), or baked or broiled chicken. You can also have two boiled eggs as a substitute for your

meat protein. Eggs are especially convenient when you are on the go. Add steamed veggies and rice, and one large salad with olive oil and apple cider vinegar for your dressing. Then add your favorite herbs. This is a guideline for your daily lunch. Make it your biggest meal. While eating, take a digestive enzyme.

- If possible, don't eat at exactly the same time every day. Eat when you are hungry! When you eat at the same time every day, the brain will send a signal to your stomach to empty, and it will seem hungry even if it is not. For instance, if you are conditioned to eat precisely at noon, even if you have had no hunger pains, your brain will still send the message that you are hungry. By eating at different times each day, you will learn to eat when you are hungry, not when the clock tells you to eat.

- Somewhere between 2:00 and 3:00 P.M., take one ounce of *Body Oxygen*™ along with another 6 ounces of *Clustered Water*™ and diet supplements.

- Throughout the afternoon or at your afternoon break, eat three fresh fruits and veggies, such as carrot sticks, celery sticks, apples, grapes, cucumbers, etc. You can eat as many fresh fruits and veggies as you like, but stay away from dressings or dips.

- Sometime before 6:00 P.M. (remember, the later you eat, the more food gets retained unburned overnight) have one cup of brown rice, a sweet potato or two red potatoes along with some lentils, red or black beans, and a piece of salmon two or three nights a week.

Season with all the onions, garlic, and a bit of extra virgin olive oil that you want. Have two servings of steamed vegetables, such as cabbage, broccoli, artichokes, beets, green beans, etc. You may use sea salt or Vege-Sal to season, but no more than 1/2 teaspoon. Along with your meal, have another salad. Eat the salad last! Take a digestive enzyme with your meal.

■ One or two cups of herbal tea without sweeteners are fine throughout the day, hot or cold.

■ Right before going to bed, eat 1/2 cup of pure oat bran with soy or rice milk. Along with the oat bran, take 2 to 4 colon cleanse capsules.

■ Fresh fruit and vegetable juices are allowed before 3:00 P.M. These must be fresh—not canned, frozen, or processed.

■ Each month plan a three-day fast!

As you can see, there are a lot of foods you can eat. But they are the right foods—pure and unprocessed. If you look at chapter 9 on the Levitical Diet, you'll see precisely what is best for you. Your body can easily digest and assimilate these foods and use them to work on healing the body, instead of expending all your energy breaking down the wrong foods. Making the daily right choices is the key to success! I believe you will choose the right foods at the right time. Ask the Holy Spirit to help you as you retrain yourself to choose wisely.

FAT-BURNING CABBAGE SOUP

Cabbage soup is a very effective burner of fat from you

system. Have as much as you desire along with a fresh salad as long as it is before 6:00 P.M.

1 head cabbage, coarsely chopped
6 cloves garlic, chopped
2 zucchini, sliced
2 carrots, chopped
2 stalks celery, chopped
2 onions, chopped
2 tomatoes, chopped
1 large chicken breast, chopped
8 cups pure water or chicken stock
2 bay leaves
½ tsp. Cayenne pepper
  Sea salt or kelp to taste

Combine all ingredients in a pot. Cover and bring to a boil. Reduce heat and simmer 20 minutes. Makes 10 servings.

OTHER DETERMINING FACTORS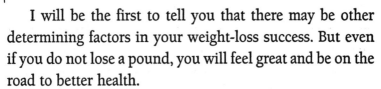

I will be the first to tell you that there may be other determining factors in your weight-loss success. But even if you do not lose a pound, you will feel great and be on the road to better health.

The following are various reasons weight loss can be difficult for some people:

- Simply overeating
- Sedentary lifestyle
- Slow metabolism, due to toxicity, leading to a sluggish digestive system

- Hypothyroidism
- Hormonal imbalance
- Various liver disorders
- Emotional disorders throwing other levels in the body out of balance
- Genetics
- *Candida Albicans*
- Adrenal disorder or failure
- Medications—Do not stop taking any of your medications without consulting your primary care physician.

For each of the above reasons, seek nutritional advice and get a plan to bring healing in those areas. God has the answer for them all.

THE ONE PERFECT DIET— THE LEVITICAL PLAN

DID YOU KNOW THAT GOD HAS PROVIDED A PLAN FOR EVERYTHING WE NEED, INCLUDING WHAT TO EAT? It's true, and God's plan is that we be submitted to Him in every area of our lives. He wants us to be free from other controls and dominion (Romans 6:14), including being in bondage to food. We've been redeemed from all bondages by the death and resurrection of Jesus Christ our Lord. I believe that He alone should have authority over our spirit, soul, and body.

We need to bring our eating under submission to God. We are spiritual beings who live in physical bodies. We are the temples of the Lord. Our body is merely a vehicle for fulfilling His purpose on the earth. Once you get that perspective, you'll eat to live, not live to eat. So before you read the following plan for eating God's way, take a moment to pray and submit yourself to God. Ask the Lord to show you areas where you can enhance your daily living by making dietary changes. He will show you, because He wants you to have victory in this area of your life.

GOD'S ANCIENT PLAN

God had a plan for healthy eating from the very beginning. Those who follow it walk in health, and those who don't are left to struggle with malnutrition, obesity, and disease. Need proof? Studies show that Israel is the healthiest nation on the earth, while the United States is ranked a dismal 96. That statistic alone should make you stop and take notice of what God has to say about your diet.

To fulfill the Word of God, the Jews observe the laws of Kashrut (keeping Kosher) as established in the Old Testament—what an awesome testimony of faithfulness and obedience to God! So many times we think of the Old Testament as a lot of do's and don'ts, but we fail to realize that God never does anything without a purpose. Those do's and don'ts have meaning! Although we will probably never know all the intricacies of the full benefits from eating God's way, I want to explore a few.

Hosea 4:6 says, "My people are destroyed from lack of knowledge." That's where most people stop reading. Let's finish the verse, though! God says, "Because you have rejected knowledge, I also reject you . . . because you have ignored the law of your God." Does that mean you're not going to heaven if you do not follow the dietary laws of the Old Testament? No, of course, not. The early church made it clear that it was not a mandatory part of the Christian faith (Acts 15). But I do believe that when we disregard the wisdom that God has already provided, we lose—in this case, our health.

Fad diets work temporarily, with an 85-percent failure rate of lasting weight loss. Starving works great until you start eating again. Exercise is fantastic, but if you don't eat right, your body will still starve for proper nutrition. This will absolutely show up in one manner or another. Everything in life is about choices, so set your will toward making right decisions and reap the wonderful rewards God has in store for you.

Psalm 103:1-5 says, "Praise the LORD, O my soul; all my inmost being, praise his holy name. Praise the LORD, O my soul, and forget not all his benefits—who forgives all your sins and heals all your diseases, who redeems your life from the pit and crowns you with love and compassion, *who satisfies your desires with good things so that your youth is renewed like the eagle's.*" So many times we only look at the fact that we want our youth renewed, and we overlook the prerequisite, which is satisfying our desires with good things. Not things that just taste good, but things that *are good* for us!

We can't separate the Word of God. For example, you may have heard someone quote, "Resist the devil, and he will flee from you" (James 4:7). That's not all that it says, though! The first half of the verse states, "Submit yourselves, then, to God." Depending upon what you quote, you get two totally different meanings. One in which you have no responsibility, and the other in which you must submit to God. We all need to submit to God's plan so that we can enjoy the true blessings of God, whether it is in spiritual warfare or in our eating. God's plan is that we treat our body as the temple of the Lord and feed it the right sustenance so that we walk in healing every day of our lives.

Blessings to all who endeavor to make lifestyle changes that will positively affect you in all you do.

Kashrut Terms

Kosher—properly prepared or ritually correct under
   Jewish law.
Milchik—food that is or contains milk or milk derivatives.
Fleischik—food that is or contains meat or meat derivatives.
Pareve—food that has none of the above properties (neu-
   tral foods such as fish, fruit, or vegetables).

Kashrut Procedures

Do not mix dairy and meat products. The traditional
Jews will not even use the same dishes or cookware; much
less eat them at the same meal.

Meat and fowl must be slaughtered correctly to be
Kosher.

Fruits and vegetables are considered pareve (neutral)
and may be served with either milk or meat foods.

Fish that has both fins and scales is considered Kosher
and pareve. However, fish is not to be cooked together
with meat.

Fundamental Rules

1. Only the meat and milk of certain animals is permitted.
   This restriction includes the flesh, organs, eggs, and
   milk of the forbidden animals.
2. Of the animals that may be eaten, the birds and mammals must be killed in accordance with the Jewish law.
3. All blood must be drained from the meat or boiled
   out of it before it is eaten.

4. Certain parts of permitted animals may not be eaten.
5. Meat (the flesh of birds and mammals) cannot be eaten with or cooked with dairy. Fish, eggs, fruits, vegetables, and grains can be eaten with either meat or dairy. (According to some views, fish may not be eaten with meat.)
6. Utensils that have come into contact with meat may not be used with dairy, and vice versa. Utensils that have come into contact with non-Kosher food may not be used with Kosher food. This applies only if the contact occurred while the food was hot.
7. Grape products made by non-Jews may not be eaten.

According to Leviticus 11:3 and Deuteronomy 14:6, you may eat any animal that has cloven hooves and chews its cud. This includes cattle, sheep, goats, buffalo, and deer. It specifically excludes the hare, pig, camel, and the rock badger (you probably won't have a problem staying away from the latter two animals).

In Leviticus 11:9 and Deuteronomy 14:9, shellfish such as lobsters, oysters, shrimp, clams, and crabs are all forbidden. Fish such as tuna, carp, salmon, and herring are all permitted.

For birds there is less criteria. Leviticus 11:13-19 and Deuteronomy 14:11-18 list birds that are forbidden but does not specify why. However, they all are birds of prey and/or scavengers, which is why the rabbis said they were set apart. Birds such as chicken, geese, ducks, and turkeys are all permitted.

SOME EXAMPLES OF NON-KOSHER FOODS ▪

Pork, rabbit, and horse meat; fowl, such as owl and stork; fish, such as catfish, eels, shellfish, shrimp, and octopus; and insects are all non-Kosher foods according to biblical definitions.

Can a Processed Food Such as Soda, Cookies, or Potato Chips Be Non-Kosher?

Yes. This is because all ingredients and sub-units in a product must conform to the dietary laws in order for the food item to be considered Kosher. Even one non-Kosher ingredient can render the entire product unsuitable. Soda may contain a flavor enhancer called castorium, which is extracted from beavers. Cookies may contain a non-Kosher emulsifier, which is derived from animal fat. Potato chips may be fried in animal oil. So read your labels carefully.

The important point is not to get into the bondage of having to look for everything marked "Kosher," but to realize that God has given us a very clear plan for the foods we should eat. For example, the laws regarding Kosher slaughter are so sanitary that Kosher butchers and slaughterhouses have been exempted from many USDA regulations.

Non-Kosher slaughterhouses often operate in a manner far different from what God intended. I know this firsthand. My husband and I visited a non-Kosher slaughterhouse to see if we were interested in raising cattle on our farm. The butcher said, chuckling to himself, "If the cow wasn't fat enough when we brought it in, we put it out back and shoot it with a few hormones to increase its weight so we can get more money." We also inquired as to how the animals were butchered. He said, "We either shoot them or knock them out with a sledgehammer." That was enough information to make our decision. Those practices are far from God's plan!

In Kosher slaughtering the method is that of slicing the throat, which causes unconsciousness within two seconds, and is widely recognized as the most humane method of slaughter possible. There is no pain or fear in the animal, with no chemical releases, whether natural or synthetic. In this method, there is also rapid and complete draining of the blood. The Bible specifies that we do not eat blood because the life of the animal is contained in the blood. This is true even for an egg that contains a blood spot when cracked.

Today we know that disease is found in the blood, and if it is not drained properly, you can ingest it into your system. To show the comparison of Kosher to non-Kosher slaughtering, look at the contrast. In the typical meat plant, many animals are brought in at one time. The animals are lined up and either shot or hit with a sledgehammer. The animals experience fear brought on by the noise of the gun, the hammer, and the animals' cries of pain. When a mammal experiences fear, adrenaline is released into its bloodstream to help it flee. As the animal is slaughtered, these hormones are released into the bloodstream and then spill over into the flesh. The blood in the organs is also spilled into the flesh. What does this mean? It means that anything previously given to the animal, such as antibiotics, hormones, or even bacteria-laden feed, will now be ingested into you as you enjoy your steak dinner.

SEPARATION OF MEAT AND DAIRY

The Torah says that meat and dairy should never be consumed together. Spiritually, the Jews believe that it is callous to take an animal's life in order to satiate their own appetites. So they don't drink milk, which represents the nurturing of animal life, when they eat meat, which represents the destruction of life.

Once again, God had a dual purpose for a waiting time between eating meat and dairy. First, there is evidence that the combining of meat and dairy interferes with digestion. It's important to realize that the key to losing weight naturally and living healthy is dependent on good digestion and the absorption of nutrients. Whatever inhibits digestion needs to be avoided.

Plus, it is no coincidence that it takes approximately three hours to digest fish and fowl and anywhere from six to eight hours to digest meat. Why extend that time with milk? No modern food preparation technique can reproduce the health benefit of the Kosher law of eating them separately.

Remember that anything from an animal is high in fat, so eat more fowl and fish and less red meat. They take less time to digest, which means more energy for you and less energy devoted to processing a large piece of meat. Stick with Kosher if possible. If Kosher is not available, go for the hormone-free.

THE EXCELLENCE OF FISH

According to Leviticus 11:9, fish is considered to be a clean food. It is naturally low in calories and rich in health-giving oils as well as essential vitamins and minerals. Fish contain important Omega-3 fatty acids, which have been proven to lower cholesterol, inhibit blood clots, lower blood pressure, and reduce the risk of heart attack and stroke.

For years cod liver oil has been used as an immune system booster and tonic to cure any number of ills. Today, medical experts are seeing the wisdom that has been in God's plan from the beginning of time. Researchers at Rutgers University have shown that fish oil is also an effective cancer fighter, reducing your risk of breast, pancreatic, lung, prostate, and colon cancers. Migraine sufferers also find great relief with Omega-3 fish oils, according to studies at the University of Cincinnati. Another study there showed that people who suffer from psoriasis were helped tremendously after taking Omega-3 fatty acid.

The best fish sources, which are naturally low in calories, are salmon, mackerel, and halibut.

Shellfish and fish without scales are high in cholesterol and considered high-stress foods. Stay away from these.

TIPS ON EATING

- Before meals, eat 4 or 5 almonds. This will help to curb your appetite by sending a signal to the brain that you are full.
- A good oat bran is a great way to end your day instead

of a heavy meal at dinner. A half-cup a day has also been proven to cut your risk of cancer by 30 percent. It is very effective in the elimination of waste from the bowels, and we know that an unhealthy eliminative system makes for a breeding ground of disease.

■ Wait 10-15 minutes before having a second helping. This is how long it takes to get the signal to the brain to tell you you're full. In doing this, you usually won't want a second helping.

■ If you can avoid it, never eat past 6:00 P.M. in the evening! The later you eat, the less likely you are of burning it up. If you are having a smoothie, the time is not important because it is easily digested and absorbed.

■ After your dinner, take a brisk walk. If your health does not allow it yet, start with walking in place for 5-10 minutes and increase as you can. If you're past that, go for it. Schedule in exercise three times a week. Remember there will never be a good time to exercise. You have to create one. At least 20-30 minutes is a good place to start. As with all changes in diet and exercise, consult with your physician first.

■ Don't drink anything with your meals. If you must drink, have water with a slice of lemon. Sodas, teas, and coffees interfere with the stomach acids and enzymes vital for digestion.

■ If you have a problem with poor digestion, try a glass of steam-distilled water with a teaspoon of raw honey, a fourth of a fresh lemon, and two tablespoons of organic apple-cider vinegar. This mixture can be taken with each meal and has been proven to increase your digestive ability. Many of those with chronic upset stomach, acid indigestion, and gaseous problems find themselves being relieved with this inexpensive home remedy.

- A study was done of men from all around the world. Surprisingly, the healthiest men over all were French! Considering the typical heavy, sauce-covered French foods, this fact is quite shocking. The three things that made the difference in their diet were the following: a little red wine, which aids in digestion; lots of fresh foods and fresh herbs; and, most important of all, they ate their salad last. The living enzymes in the fresh vegetable eaten last works to break down all the other foods just eaten. It is an excellent palate cleanser, and because of that, it helps you to make the right choice in not choosing a dessert. With all your food being broken down more efficiently, you get better absorption of all your nutrients, you feel better, and you have more energy. It is not abnormal to have your salad served last in a European country, so next time you're dining out, go the European way. Eat your salad last!

- Remember: the ball of your fist is the size of your stomach when it is empty. Open up your palm. That should be the portion size you eat at each meal. More than that at a time, and you are overeating!

TIPS ON FOODS

- Eat as many *fresh fruits and vegetables* a day as possible. By eating five per day, according to Johns Hopkins

University, you can cut your risk of cancer by 30 percent and lower your systolic blood pressure by 5.5 points and the diastolic pressure by 3.0 points. Their researchers concluded that you could reduce your risk of heart disease by 15 percent and the risk of a stroke by 27 percent.

■ Researchers at Loma Linda University in California have shown scientifically that Kyolic® (a brand of garlic capsules found in any health food store) reduces the dangerous LDL levels of the blood and increases the beneficial HDL levels. A study in India showed that garlic has the ability to reduce blood clotting as well as serve as an anti-cancer agent.

■ Go to your local health food store and get a good powdered kelp to use for your seasoning. This is a great additive to your food as well as a plus to the thyroid, which controls your entire metabolism. A liquid bladder wrack—an old herbal remedy used for low thyroid—is also excellent when on a weight-loss program. It's very natural to the body and excellent for weight loss by speeding up the metabolism with no harmful side effects.

■ A good rule of thumb is to stay away from processed foods. Then you don't have to be concerned about those hidden ingredients labeled as "natural flavoring." Try to eat foods that are as close to the way that God created them—chemical free!

■ Water is vitally important to your body. Drink half your weight in ounces daily. Adding more water to your diet will make a big difference in your weight loss and health level, as well as change.

- Think about sprouting at home. It's easy, it's fun, it's cheap, and it tastes good! Even the kids love them and love to grow them! They're great on sandwiches and salads, and they can be used as snacks as well. The rewards are great. They are loaded with trace minerals that are not so easily found in other foods. You can get everything you need at your local health food store to sprout.

- Go for foods rich in color! Stay away from the white deadly things! White sugar, white flour, white salt, even white potatoes. Choose red potatoes instead of white. Choose a dark lettuce or spinach instead of iceberg.

- Go for Bible snacks instead of the processed foods. Fresh fruits, fresh veggies, nuts, raisins, granolas, yogurts, unrefined crackers, and flat breads—get creative! Genesis 43:11 specifically mentions pistachios and almonds. That's interesting in that those are particularly low in fat and calories. Nuts in general are a great snack food, with the exception of peanuts, which are really not a nut! Nuts are naturally rich in zinc, copper, iron, calcium, magnesium, and phosphorus, as well as being high in protein. Dr. Walter Troll of New York University says that nuts are among the top cancer-fighting foods in the world, containing cancer blockers. Nuts also help to keep blood sugar levels steady so you don't get those bothersome hunger pangs that can lead you to grab the first snack you can find, which is normally high in sugar and carbohydrates.

■ Yogurt, or fermented milk, isn't mentioned in the Bible, but according to history we know that it was a mainstay at that time. Yogurt has been attributed to longevity in many civilizations. It is the ideal diet food for folks who want to add flavor and health benefits to their diet. Be sure not to get the yogurt with artificial sweeteners or with added sugars. Yogurt is a natural antibiotic that keeps your digestive system healthy by replacing the good flora in the intestinal track. This is needed for a healthy immune system. You can use yogurt in a variety of ways with salad dressings. It's a healthy snack—my favorite is my *Creation's Bounty* Shake with yogurt in the mornings!Those who are lactose-intolerant typically do fine with a good yogurt.

■ Extra virgin olive oil is by far the best oil you can use! It has been proven to be the healthiest for your heart as well as lowering your cholesterol level instead of clogging your arteries the way the saturated fats found in your typical grocery store oils and margarinated butter does. It is far more versatile and can be used for just about anything. Medicinally speaking, olive oil has proven to be a natural antibiotic as well as antiviral. It tastes great and is good for you!

PRACTICAL APPLICATION

Putting the Levitical Diet into your daily living is actually very easy once you get in the swing of things. The important key is to get the body back into a place of homeostasis, which is a happy, healthy body, and the proper foods will make a world of difference. The rewards of healthy living, an energetic body, and sound, clear thinking will cause you to never want to turn back.

Remember that God's way works!

FOODS THAT SUPERCHARGE YOUR MIND AND BODY

THE SCIENTIFIC EVIDENCE IS OVERWHELMING: IF YOU WANT TO FEEL GREAT ALL THE TIME, YOU NEED TO MAKE CERTAIN YOU ARE EATING A HEALTHY, ENERGY-PACKED DIET that balances your intake of antioxidants, calcium, complex carbohydrates, essential fatty acids, and proteins. It is important that those foods deliver plenty of fiber, vitamins, and minerals. For most of us it involves moving away from a diet high in processed food, sugar, fat, and meat to a diet that revolves around whole grains, fresh vegetables, and fresh fruits.

Energy foods benefit the mind as well as the body. What you eat shapes the health of your cells and organs as well as their ability to function and repair themselves. Nutritional deficiencies cause a breakdown in the building blocks for your body's compounds, hormones, and enzymes. *All* the basic functions of your body, including your brain, are dependent upon an adequate supply of nutrition, and they operate only as efficiently as they are healthy.

SUPER COMPLEX CARBOHYDRATES

Complex carbohydrates are derived from carbon, hydrogen, and oxygen. Sugar, starch, and cellulose are carbohydrates. They are a major source of energy in our diet and are found in grains, legumes, fruits, vegetables, sugar, and alcohol. They have beneficial effects on the way we absorb and use our nutrients.

You need to keep in mind that some carbohydrates release their energy slowly and provide long-lasting sustenance. These are the ones you want—primarily the brown grains, fruits, or leafy green foods with all their fiber intact. One value of the fiber is that it prolongs the carbohydrate's energy release for hours after you've eaten.

Then there are the carbohydrates that release quickly— the refined white starchy foods, sugars, and alcohol. They deliver a burst of energy that gets you through the moment but leaves you exhausted in the long run. Sugar is the most addictive substance in our diets, and food manufacturers know it. You'll find sugar in almost every processed or packaged food, and the cumulative effect is reflected in bulging waistlines and poor health. You have to cut out the heavy intake of sugar.

Excellent carbohydrate sources are vegetables of all kinds (raw whenever possible), fruits, legumes, milk, whole grains, and whole wheat pasta. The good news is that foods containing complex carbohydrates, such as bread and pasta, are usually rich in vitamins, minerals, and trace elements.

SUPER PROTEINS

As the famed building blocks of the body, proteins consist of long, folded chains of amino acids. You need them for building and repairing body tissues, and for producing hormones, enzymes, and nerve chemicals. They are vital for sustaining a healthy immune system and need to be taken in daily, because your body cannot store them.

While it is well known that lean meat, fish, full-fat dairy products, and eggs are excellent sources of protein, did you know that plant foods contain protein and that vegetables, whole grains, nuts, seeds, and legumes are all good sources? For example, ounce for ounce, steak contains less protein than soy flour. If possible, stay away from foods that have been smoked, are high in fat, or that contain chemical preservatives (such as most sausages).

SUPER ANTIOXIDANTS

I addressed the role antioxidants have in our body's detoxification process on page 106. Antioxidants, such as beta-carotene, Vitamins A, E, and especially C, and selenium, neutralize the free radicals that are produced in the process of metabolism in our bodies. They protect our cells against damage and mutation. The more antioxidants we get in our diets, the more we are able to stop these damaging effects.

The main source of antioxidants is fruits, vegetables, nuts, whole grains, and cold-pressed plant oils.

SUPER ESSENTIAL FATTY ACIDS

Fat is as essential to our diets as any other component, despite the constant warnings we have heard about it. Fat helps to build cell membranes in every cell in the body. Good fats affect the brain so much that every area of sensory and motor skills either improves or declines through what you eat. Fats ensure that the nervous system functions properly.

While it's true that we eat far too many saturated (usually solid at room temperature) and hydrogenated fats from sources such as meat, dairy products, margarine, cooking oils, and packaged food, certain fats are needed for good health. Unsaturated fats (usually soft at room temperature and often called oils) are divided into monounsaturated fats and polyunsaturated fats.

Monounsaturated fats appear to provide some protection from heart disease and are the best for cooking, as they do not tend to undergo chemical changes when they are heated. Polyunsaturated fats are prone to changes when they are exposed to light, heat, the air, and other chemicals. If they are processed, such as in the manufacture of margarine, chemical changes can occur, leading to the production of "trans-fats." These are fats that the body cannot easily break down and often lead to blocked arteries and heart disease.

Two polyunsaturated fatty acids, linoleic acid and alpha-linolenic acid, are known as essential fatty acids because our body does not produce them. These come mainly from the Omega family of fats. Good Omega-3 fats include: flaxseed, hemp seed, pumpkin seed, soy, walnuts, leafy green vegetables, fish oil, salmon, trout, mackerel, herring, blue fin, sardines, anchovies, and albacore tuna. Good Omega-6 fats include: walleye, carp, pike, haddock, sesame oil, borage seed oil, evening primrose oil, unrefined sunflower oil, walnuts, chicken, rice bran, black current seeds, fresh unroasted and unsalted nuts and seeds, and eggs. Good Omega-9 fats include: olive oil, avocados, and meats.

SUPER CALCIUM

From the time you were young, you were told that calcium is crucial for building and maintaining healthy bones and teeth. You may not have been told that it also plays an important role in the function of nerves, muscles, enzymes, and hormones. Calcium normalizes the contraction and relaxation of the heart muscles and protects against osteoporosis, rickets, and osteomalacia.

Most plant foods contain calcium—spinach, watercress, parsley, dried figs, nuts, seeds, molasses, seaweed, dried beans, broccoli, and soy are all rich suppliers. Milk, eggs, salmon, and sardines are good calcium sources. Tofu delivers a whopping four times more calcium than whole milk, ounce for ounce.

SUPER VITAMINS

Vitamins constitute one of the major groups of nutrients, which are food substances necessary for growth and health. They regulate chemical reactions through which the body converts food into energy and living tissues. Of the 13 vitamins we need, 5 are produced by the body itself. Of those 5, only 3 can be produced in sufficient quantities to meet the body's needs. Therefore, vitamins must be supplied in a person's daily diet.

We tend to think that any vitamin will do, but this is not the case. Every vitamin has a specific function that nothing else can replace. And, if you lack any vitamin, it can actually hinder the function of another. Vitamin deficiency diseases, such as beriberi, pellagra, rickets, or scurvy, are the result of an ongoing lack of a vitamin.

A well-balanced diet from all the basic food groups is the best way to obtain these essential vitamins. If you take supplements, always take a food-based multivitamin capsule as well as specific nutrients to help them work more effectively. Do not exceed the doses printed on the packaging.

VITAMIN	PURPOSE	SOURCE
A (Retinol)	Promotes healthy skin, bones, teeth, gums, eyes, urinary tract, and lining of the nervous, respiratory, and digestive systems.	Full-fat dairy products, fish liver oil, liver, eggs, butter, sweet potatoes, yellow and green vegetables.
B1 (Thiamine)	Required for carbohydrate metabolism and the release of energy from food. Helps your heart and nervous system function properly.	Whole grains and whole-grain breads and cereals, nuts, sunflower seeds, peas, potatoes, and most vegetables.
B2 (Riboflavin)	Promotes healthy hair, skin, nails, and tissue repair. Helps body cells use oxygen.	Liver, full-fat milk, cheese, eggs, liver, fish, poultry, almonds, and leafy green vegetables.
B3 (Niacin)	Helps maintain healthy skin and digestive tract and hormone production. Essential for cell metabolism and absorption of carbohydrates.	Lean meat, liver, whole grain and whole grain products, eggs, milk, nuts, potatoes, avocados, and soy flour.
B5 (Panthothenic acid)	Promotes healthy skin, hormone production, muscles, and nerves. Helps convert carbohydrates, fats, and proteins into energy.	Nuts, eggs, meat, whole-grain cereals, legumes, and green vegetables.
B6 (Pyridoxine)	For healthy teeth and gums, blood vessels, nervous and immune systems, and red blood cells.	Whole-grain cereals, liver, poultry, fish, meat, eggs, most vegetables, and sunflower seeds.
B12	Helps prevent infection and anemia through the proper development of red blood cells. Aids the nervous system.	Fish, dairy products, meats, whole-grain breads, and eggs.

VITAMIN	PURPOSE	SOURCE
BIOTIN	Assists the circulatory system and promotes healthy skin.	Eggs, liver, nuts, kidneys, and most fresh vegetables.
C (Ascorbic acid)	Vital for the immune system as well as for skin, bone, teeth, cartilage formation, and for wound healing.	Citrus fruits, tomatoes, raw cabbage, sweet potatoes, cauliflower, leafy green vegetables, peppers, broccoli, potatoes, strawberries, and cantaloupe.
D (Cholecalciferol)	Helps calcium to be utilized for bones and promotes a healthy heart and nervous system.	Fish liver oils, salmon, tuna, leafy green vegetables, mushrooms, eggs, full-fat milk, butter, and sunlight.
E (Tocopherol)	Promotes healthy cell membranes by helping to prevent the oxidation of polyunsaturated fatty acids in those membranes and other body structures. Aids fertility, stamina, and combating changes of old age.	Leafy green vegetables, wheat germ oil, olive oil, eggs, tomatoes, soy beans, brown rice, fresh nuts and seeds, and whole grains.
FOLIC ACID	Needed for the production of red blood cells and helps in the prevention of anemia, heart disease, and congenital abnormalities.	Leafy green vegetables, fruit, whole grains, liver, meat, poultry, fish, and full-fat milk.
K	Needed for normal blood clotting, healthy bones, and teeth.	Leafy green vegetables, cheese, liver, eggs, fish, full-fat milk, safflower oil, kelp, and raspberry leaf tea.

MINERAL	PURPOSE	SOURCE
CALCIUM	For healthy bones, teeth, muscles, and essential for nerve message transmission.	Dairy products, soy (such as tofu), nuts, seeds, dried beans, leafy green vegetables, broccoli, and salmon.
CHROMIUM	Promotes the correct blood sugar levels and helps lower cholesterol levels.	Whole grains, brown rice, eggs, molasses, red meat, wine, bananas, lettuce, oranges, strawberries, apples, potatoes, parsnips.
COPPER	For the blood, bones, and nervous system.	Legumes, nuts, olives, and seafood.
IODINE	Regulates the thyroid gland.	All seafood, kelp, samphire, and iodized salt.
IRON	Essential in the formation of red blood cells and prevention of anemia.	Liver, red meat, eggs, dried fruit, asparagus, legumes, green vegetables, oatmeal, walnuts, sunflower seeds, and mushrooms.
MAGNESIUM	Essential for nerve and muscle function and maintaining blood pressure.	Dark leafy green vegetables, citrus fruit, nuts, whole grains, seeds, raisins, garlic, onions, potatoes, and chicken.
POTASSIUM	Needed for healthy bones, brain function, water balance, and fighting fatigue and muscle weakness.	Salmon, lamb, and all vegetables and fruits, particularly bananas, watermelon, and potatoes.
SELENIUM	Detoxifies arsenic and mercury and fights infections.	Whole grains, brown rice, Brazil nuts, seafood, eggs, and tomatoes.
SODIUM	Helps regulate the water in the body.	Salt and salty foods.
ZINC	Fights against infections and heavy metals, repairs wounds, and helps normal sexual functions. Needed for immune systems and enzyme production.	Seeds, nuts, whole grains, meat, eggs, brown rice, and berries.

The Value of Salt in Your Diet

Table salt, as we commonly know it, truly deserves the horrible reputation it has gotten over the past twenty years and should not be used. Today, every common table salt sold is artificial. It is responsible for causing high blood pressure and heart problems.

But it is a mistake to confuse table salt with sea salt, which contains many health-promoting minerals such as magnesium, calcium, potassium, sodium, chloride, sulfate, phosphate, and many trace minerals. These trace minerals are absolutely vital in the electrolytic activity of the whole body, and without them you simply cannot function.

And without salt you can't make adequate amounts of HCL (stomach acid), and in this weakened digestive state you can't absorb the minerals that are vital for activating enzymes and other important metabolic functions. Salt is also needed to maintain water balance within cells, control pH levels, and emulsify fats and fat-soluble vitamins. If you are avoiding salts you may experience low blood pressure, dizziness, chronic fatigue, poor digestion, and hypo-adrenal function.

Instead of avoiding salt, which is a healthy nutrient our bodies need, you need to go to a health food store and pick up sea salt.

Healthy Snacks to Keep on Hand

- Fresh fruit
- Seeds and nuts

- Carrot sticks and celery stalks
- Half an avocado with a squeeze of lemon and ground pepper
- Apples and small squares of cheese or cottage cheese
- Salads
- Boiled eggs
- Raisins
- Mashed bananas sprinkled with cinnamon
- Applesauce
- Live yogurt
- 100 percent rye crackers
- Chinese rice crackers
- 100 percent fruit chewy bars

INEXPENSIVE HEALTH FOODS

- Beans and lentils
- Vegetables of all kinds
- Fruits in season
- Oily fish, especially salmon
- Water
- Whole grains
- Lean meat, especially chicken

SUPER FOODS

- Red grapes—considered a better antioxidant than green grapes and contains anthrocyanins, which are thought to decrease the stickiness of blood platelets and reduce the likelihood of blood clots. They also contain reservatol, which lowers blood cholesterol and may inhibit the formation of cancer cells.

- Carrots—rich in carotenes and an excellent source of chromium and fiber. Beta-carotene may help prevent cancer of the lungs, cervix, and gastrointestinal tract. Carrots also give your immunity system a boost.
- Oranges and grapefruit—high Vitamin C content helps to maintain healthy blood cells and may increase resistance to viral infections. Vitamin C may also help lower blood cholesterol and protect against breast cancer.
- Beets—rich in folic acid, iron, and magnesium. Have been used to relieve all chronic illnesses, particularly those of the blood and immune system. Thought to also help the body fight cancer.
- Cranberry—long used to relieve urinary-tract infections because it contains a phytochemical that prevents harmful bacteria from sticking to the bladder wall. In addition, it has powerful antioxidant effects that may improve cardiovascular health.

NINE CANCER-FIGHTERS

- Broccoli
- Cauliflower
- Grapefruit
- Licorice Root
- Tomato (raw)
- Garlic
- Cabbage
- Concord Grapes
- Green Tea

SUBSTITUTES FOR ADDICTIONS

- Sugar—stevia fructose, barley malt, and molasses are far better. Sweeten desserts with stewed fruit. Use a little raw honey. Finely chopped dried fruit or mashed bananas works well on cereals, porridge, yogurt, cakes, and pie bases.
- Coffee—barley, chicory, or dandelion (raises blood pressure) coffee.
- Chocolate—low-sugar muesli bar, carob bar, fruit bar, dried fruit.
- Strong tea—weak tea, whether green, ginger, mint, or fruit.
- Colas—find a delicious herbal drink or a juice mixed with sparkling water or ginseng colas from health food stores.
- Alcohol—a spicy tomato juice, sparkling water with ice and a slice of lemon, or an herbal drink.

FINE-TUNE FOR YOUR SPECIFIC NEEDS

*They found an Egyptian in a field
and brought him to David.
They gave him water to drink
and food to eat—part of a cake
of pressed figs and two cakes of raisins.
He ate and was revived, for he had not
eaten any food or drunk any water
for three days and three nights*

1 SAMUEL 30:12-12

NATURE'S PRESCRIPTIONS FOR FEELING GREAT

I BELIEVE THAT GOD HAS MADE HEALING AVAILABLE TO EVERY PERSON. His first way is divine health, which occurs whenever a person is walking daily in God's plan and experiencing a wholeness of spirit, soul, and body. Second, God brings healing to individuals who experience health challenges and require His direct touch in a miraculous way that may manifest in an instantaneous healing or recovery manifesting itself physically. I have personally been healed in this dramatic manner, and I have prayed with others who were healed directly as we prayed. Third, God placed herbs, minerals, and vitamins for us to understand and utilize to maintain health and regain health. He has instructed man through His Word on how to utilize these for our personal wellness. I have written this guide to help make you aware of possible natural products that may help. Fourth, there's medicine. I thank God for Godly medical doctors. God in His grace has made provision for every situation.

Most of the substances mentioned in this booklet can be obtained through a health food store without a prescription. But self-care and self-diagnosis should never be a substitute for appropriate diagnosis by a trained health professional. I cannot overstate this.

HERBS

For thousands of years, not just hundreds of years, herbs have provided a constant supply of healing agents to people. Whether from the roots, leaves, bark, flowers, or berries of plants, herbs have been scientifically proven to be nature's pharmaceutical agents as well as very effective in the prevention of illness. They are powerful, though usually gentle, and are a safe and natural alternative to drugs when used properly. You will find them packaged as teas, salves, tinctures, capsules, tablets, and concentrated extracts. Always follow the manufacturer's advice regarding the dosage.

In the following chart you may find natural alternatives to drugs for some of the most common problems faced by mankind. If you do use any of the following, please refer to the following guidelines.

1. Consult a physician if you have an illness. Naturopaths, Holistic M.D.s, Osteopaths, Chiropractors, and Natural Health specialists are also available.

2. If you are using a prescribed medication, you must ask your physician prior to discontinuing any medication.

3. Talk with your physician prior to starting any natural alternative that you might use from this book.

4. Remember everyone needs a total health plan, including diet, supplementation, life-style factors, and spiritual factors.

5. These statements have not been evaluated by the Food and Drug Administration and are not intended to diagnose, treat, cure, or prevent any disease or illness.

CONDITIONS	PRESCRIPTIONS	ALTERNATIVES
ANGINA	Nitroglycerin	Carnitine, CoQ10, Magnesium, Hawthorne, and Khella, Hyperberic Oxygen, *Body Oxygen*™, *Clustered Water*™
ASTHMA HAY FEVER	Seldane, Bronchodilators, Albuterol, Cromolyn, Xanthine Preparations	Local Bee Pollen, Garlic, Mullein, Fenugreek, Thyme, Flaxseed Oil, *Body Oxygen*™, *Body Oxygen Spray*™
GOUT	Indomethacin	Black Cherry Juice
HERPES	Acyclovir, Zovirax	Melissa Cream, *Body Oxygen*™, *Olive Leaf Extract*™, *Oxygen Bath*™, *Clustered Water*™
PEPTIC ULCERS	Antibiotics, Tagamet, Zantac	*Body Oxygen*™, Goat's Milk
PROSTATE	Proscar	Zinc, Saw Palmetto Berry Extract, Pumpkin Seeds
LOW IRON	Iron Injections	Black Strap Molasses, Liquid Minerals, Dandelion Root
LYME	Antibiotics	Green Drink, *Body Oxygen*™, *Clustered Water*™
EDEMA	Lasix, Diazide	*Clustered Water*™, Butchers Broom, Horsetail, Parsley
WEIGHT LOSS	Phenylpropanolamine (PPA)	Fiber, Green Tea, Kola Nut, Fo Ti, Chick Weed, Spirulina, Ma Huang, *Body Oxygen*™, Bladder Wrack
NURSING	Hormone Injections	Fiber Yeast, *Body Oxygen*™, Fenugreek
SEXUAL	Viagra	Yohimbi, Wild Oats, Avina Sativa, *Clustered Water*™

CONDITIONS	PRESCRIPTIONS	ALTERNATIVES
ACNE	Retin-A, Tetracycline	Tea Tree Oil (external); Calendula, Burdock, Yellow Dock
ALLERGIES	Synthetic Antihistamines	Fenugreek, Thyme, Bee Pollen, B-Complex, *Body Oxygen*™
ANXIETY	Ativan, Xanax, Klonopin	Hops, Kava-Kava, Valerian, St. John's Wort, *Body Oxygen*™, B-Complex, Sam-E, Melissa, *Calcium/ Magnesium Complex*™
ARTHRITIC PAIN	Tylenol, other NSAIDS (nonsteroidal anti-inflammatory drugs). Aleve.	Cayenne (external); Celery Seed, Ginger, Turmeric, MSM, *Body Oxygen*™, Flax Seed Oil, *Clustered Water*™, Glucosamine
ATHLETE'S FOOT	Griseofulvin	Tea Tree Oil (external); Garlic, *Colloidal Silver*™, Hydrogen Peroxide
BOILS	Erythromycin	Tea Tree Oil, Slippery Elm (both external); Burdock, Charcoal Poultice, Yellow Dock
BPH (Benign Prostatic Hyperplasia)	Hytrin, Proscar	Saw Palmetto, Evening Primrose
BODY ODOR, PERSPIRATION	Commercial Deodorants, Antiperspirants	Coriander, Sage, Tea Tree Oil, Chlorophyll
BRONCHITIS	Atropine	Echinacea, Garlic, Plural Root, Mullein, *Body Oxygen*™, Olive Leaf
BRUISES	Analgesics	Arnica, St. John's Wort, Yarrow, Plantain (all external); Vitamin K, BioFlavonoids

CONDITIONS	PRESCRIPTIONS	ALTERNATIVES
BURNS	Silvadene Cream	Aloe (external); *Hydrogen Peroxide Gel*™, *Colloidal Silver*™
COLDS	Decongestants	Echinacea, Ginger, Lemon Balm, Garlic, Olive Leaf, *Body Oxygen*™, *Colloidal Silver*™
CONSTIPATION	Laxative	Flaxseed, Psyllium, Flora Fit, *Body Oxygen*™, Senna, Cascara Sagrada, Slippery Elm
CUTS, SCRAPES, ABSCESSES	Topical Antibiotics	Tea Tree Oil, Calendula, Plantain (all external); *Body Oxygen*™, *Colloidal Silver*™
MILD DEPRESSION	Prozac, Elavil, Trazodone, Zoloft	St. John's Wort, Melissa, *Body Oxygen*™, L-Taurine
DIARRHEA	Imodium, Lomotil	Bilberry, Raspberry, Olive Leaf, Charcoal, Slippery Elm
DYSMENORRHEA (painful menstruation)	Naprosyn	Kava-Kava, Raspberry, Valerian, *Body Oxygen*™, Lavender Oil
EARACHE	Antibiotics	Echinacea, Garlic, Mullein, *Colloidal Silver*™
ECZEMA (itchy rash)	Corticosteroids	Chamomile, Evening Primrose Oil
ATOPIC ECZEMA (allergy-related rash)	Corticosteroids, Sedatives, Antihistamines	Evening Primrose, B-Complex, *Body Oxygen*™, *Colloidal Minerals*™
FLU	Tylenol, over the counter	Echinacea, Elderberry, Bone Set, *Body Oxygen*™, Olive Leaf
GAS	Mylanta, Gaviscon, Simethicone	Dill, Fennel, Peppermint, Charcoal, Ginger, Marshmallow Root

CONDITIONS	PRESCRIPTIONS	ALTERNATIVES
GINGIVITIS (gum inflammation)	Peridex	Chamomile, Echinacea, Sage, *Hydrogen Peroxide Gel*™
HALITOSIS (bad breath)	Listerine	Cardamom, Parsley, Peppermint, Chlorophyll
HAY FEVER	Antihistamines, Decongestants	Stinging Nettle, CoQ 10, *Body Oxygen*™, Bee Pollen, Raw Honey
HEADACHE	Aspirin, other NSAIDS (nonsteroidal anti-inflammatory drugs)	Peppermint (external); Feverfew, White Willow, Lavender, *Body Oxygen*™
HEARTBURN	Pepto-Bismol, Tums	Angelica, Chamomile, Peppermint, *Body Oxygen*™, HCL
HEMORRHOIDS	Tucks	Plantain, Witch Hazel (both external); White Oak Bark, Comphrey Root Poultice, Elderberry Root Poultice
HEPATITIS	Interferon	Dandelion, Milk Thistle, Turmeric, Red Clover, Sam-E, *Body Oxygen*™, CoQ 10, MSM, Panothenic Acid, Alpha Lipoic Acid, Licorice Root
HIGH BLOOD PRESSURE	ACE Inhibitors	Cayenne, Green Tea, Olive Leaf
HYPERTHYROIDISM	Beta-Andergenic Blockers	Silver Creek Labs Multi-Vitamin, B-Complex, Brewer's Yeast, Essential Fatty Acids
HYPOTHYROIDISM	Thyroxine	Bladder wrack, Kelp, L-Tyrosine, Raw Thyroid Glandular
HIGH CHOLESTEROL	Mevacor	Garlic, Slippery Elm, Hawthorne Berry, B-Complex, *Body Oxygen*™

CONDITIONS	PRESCRIPTIONS	ALTERNATIVES
HIVES	Benadryl	Stinging Nettle, Ephedrine
INDIGESTION	Antacids, Raglan	Chamomile, Ginger, Peppermint, *Body Oxygen™*, Marshmallow Root
INSOMNIA	Halcyon, Ativan	Chamomile, Hops, Lemon Balm, Valerian, Kava-Kava, Evening Primrose Oil, *Magnesium/ Calcium™*, Vitamin C
IRREGULARITY	Metamucil	Flaxseed, Plantain, Senna
LOW BACK PAIN	Aspirin, Analgescis	Cayenne (external); Thyme Fever Few, Panothenic Acid
MALE PATTERN BALDNESS	Rogaine	Saw Palmetto, Folic Acid
MIGRAINE	Cafergot, Sumatriptan, Verapamil	Fever Few, Vaterian Root, *Body Oxygen™*
MOTION SICKNESS	Dramamine	Ginger
NAIL FUNGUS	Ketoconazole	Tea Tree Oil (external); *Olive Leaf Extract™*
NIGHT BLINDNESS	Vitamin A	Bilberry, Blueberry
PMS	NSAIDS (nonsteroidal anti-inflammatory drugs), Diuretics, Analgesics	Chaste Tree, Folic Acid, Evening Primrose Oil, *Body Oxygen™*
RHINITIS (nasal inflammation)	Cromolyn, Vancenase	Echinacea, *Colloidal Silver™*
SHINGLES	Acyclovir	Cayenne (external); Lemon Balm, Melissa
SPRAIN	NSAIDS (nonsteroidal anti-inflammatory drugs)	Arnica, Calendula, *Body Oxygen™*, MSM, White Willow
STRESS	Diazepam	Kava-Kava, Valerian, *Body Oxygen*, Vitamin C, *Calcium/Magnesium Complex™*

CONDITIONS	PRESCRIPTIONS	ALTERNATIVES
TINNITUS (ringing in the ears)	Steroids	Ginkgo, *Body Oxygen*™, Hydrogen Peroxide Bath
TOOTHACHE	NSAIDS (nonsteroidal anti-inflammatory drugs)	Cloves, Willow, Charcoal Poultice, Black Walnut Hull
URINARY TRACT INFECTIONS	Sulfa Drugs	Cranberry, Stinging Nettle
VAGINITIS	Clindamycin, Flagyl	Garlic, Goldenseal
STREPTOCOCCUS	Augmentin	OregonGrape, *Colloidal Silver*™, Olive Leaf
PARASITES		Worm Wood, Black Walnut Hull, Cloves, *Body Oxygen*, Flora Fit, *Clustered Water*™
ULCERS	Zantac, Tagamet	Cats Claw, *Body Oxygen*™, Goat's Milk

ESSENTIAL MEDICINAL HERBS

1. Aloe Vera. Internal and external; laxative, antiulcer, immune, antiviral, aids.
2. Bilberry. Diabetic retinopathy, macular degeneration, cataract, glaucoma, varicose veins.
3. Bromilene. Inflammation, sports injuries, respiratory tract infections, menstrual cramps.
4. Burdock. Mild detoxifier, promotes the production of urine and sweat.
5. Chamomile. Relaxing tea that aids digestion and the production of urine.
6. Dandelion Root. Liver disorders, water retention, obesity. Good source of potassium.
7. Dong Quai. Menopausal symptoms, premenstrual symptoms.
8. Echinacea. Viral infections, impaired immune functions, wound healing.
9. Ephedra. Asthma, hay fever, common cold, weight loss.
10. Fennel. Relieves cramps and gas.
11. Feverfew. Migraine headaches, arthritis, fever, inflammation.
12. Garlic. Infections, elevated cholesterol levels, high blood pressure, diabetes.
13. Ginger. Nausea and vomiting with pregnancy, motion sickness, arthritis.
14. Ginkgo Biloba. Decreased blood supply to brain, senility, ringing ears, dizziness, impotence, varicose veins, Alzheimer's disease.

15. Ginseng. Recovery from illness, stress, fatigue, diabetes, improvement of mental and physical performance, sexual function.
16. Golden Seal. Parasitic infections of gastronomical tract, infection of mucous membrane, inflammation of gallbladder.
17. Gotu Kola. Cellulite, wound healing, varicose veins, scleroderma.
18. Gugulipid. Elevated cholesterol and triglyceride levels, arteriosclerosis, hypothyroidism.
19. Hawthorn. Arteriosclerosis, high blood pressure, congestive heart failure, angina.
20. Hops. Cramps and gas.
21. Lapacho. Infections, *Candida Albicans*.
22. Licorice Root. Peptic ulcer, premenstrual tension syndrome, low adrenal function, viral infections.
23. Linseeds. Boost the liver with Omega-3 oils.
24. Lobelia. Smoking deterrent, expectorant in asthma, bronchitis, and pneumonia.
25. Milk Thistle or Silymarin. Liver disorders, hepatitis, cirrhosis of the liver, psoriasis.
26. Psyllium. Cholesterol.
27. Rosemary. Migraines, tension headaches, exhaustion, and fatigue.
28. Sage. Liver stimulant to promote the flow of bile.
29. Sarsaparilla. Psoriasis, Eczema, general tonic.
30. Saw Palmetto. Prostate enlargement.
31. Slippery Elm. Gentle laxative.
32. St. John's Wort. Depression, anxiety, sleep disturbance,

aids in healing nerve damage, anti-viral.

33. Tea Tree Oil. Topical antiseptic, athlete's foot, boils, wound healing.

34. Turmeric. Inflammation, arthritis, liver, gallbladder.

35. Uva Ursi. Urinary track infections, water retention.

36. Valerian. Insomnia, anxiety, high blood pressure, intestinal spasm.

SPECIFIC CONCERNS REGARDING HERBS

The following are recommendations on the use of herbs from the book *Using Herbal Alternative* by Dr. James A. Duke and the book *What the Labels Won't Tell You* by Logan Chamberlain, Ph.D.

Make sure of the diagnosis. Self-diagnosis is a risky business and best left to well-trained physicians. Once you're confident of a diagnosis, then discuss with your physician how to treat it: drugs, herbs, some combination of the two, or any of the foregoing plus diet, exercise, and lifestyle changes.

Watch out for side effects. If you have an unpleasant reaction to an herb, such as dizziness, nausea, or headache, cut back on your dosage or stop taking the herb. Listen to your body.

Beware of interactions. Pharmaceutical medications sometimes interact badly with one another and with certain foods. The same goes for herbal medicines. Always be particularly careful when taking more than one drug or herb or a combination of a drug and herb. Consult your physician or pharmacist.

If you're pregnant, take special precautions. As a general rule, you shouldn't take herbs while you're pregnant unless you discuss your selections with your obstetrician, because certain herbs can increase the risk of miscarriage.

VITAMINS AND MINERALS

The entirety of this book has emphasized the importance of the supply of the essential nutrients that your body requires through a healthy, balanced diet. While I say that, I also recognize that there are a host of reasons to supplement your diet with vitamins and minerals. Unfortunately, in today's society even when we eat the right foods we may not be getting the right nutrients in our food!

Crops are not rotated, and today's chemical fertilizers have not been replenishing the ground with the vital minerals such as magnesium and selenium. Harvesting is often too early, and a wide variety of chemicals are used to get crops to market in sellable condition for optimal sales. Vitamins are lost when food is stored. Bottom line: Your food is depleted of nutrients, vitamins, and minerals, and so are you! We do not get the minerals or vitamins we need on a daily basis through what we eat.

Because of that we must take extra supplements! Most do not realize that if you are lacking in minerals, very few of the nutrients you ingest will be absorbed, so a liquid mineral supplement is mandatory in most cases. Also, when you are under stress at work or home, making a move, changing jobs, sick, etc., all your water-soluble vitamins are depleted within one to two hours! Stress takes a special toll on the "B's" that provide the body's peace and much more. A "B" complex, food-based vitamin will help.

Vitamins are a group of organic compounds that are essential for normal growth, development, and metabolism. They are produced by living material, plants and animals, as compared to minerals that come from the soil. Insufficient supplies of any of the vitamins results in specific deficiency diseases. Vitamins function along with enzymes in chemical reactions necessary for human bodily function, including energy production. Vitamins and enzymes also work together to act as a catalyst in speeding up the making or breaking of chemical bonds that join molecules together.

Vitamins are classified into two groups. Fat-soluble vitamins (A, D, E, and K) dissolve in fat and are stored in the fatty parts of the liver and other tissues. Water-soluble vitamins (the Bs and C) dissolve in water and are not stored by the body to any great extent.

Minerals function, along with vitamins, as components of body enzymes. Minerals are needed for proper composition of teeth and bone and blood. They are important to the production of hormones and enzymes and in the creation of antibodies. Some minerals (calcium, potassium, and sodium) have electrical charges that act as a magnet to attract other electrically charged substances to form complex molecules, conduct electrical impulses along nerves, and transport substances in and out of the cells.

Deficiencies of minerals are more prevalent than deficiencies of vitamins. If you are a vegetarian, elderly, on a low-calorie diet, taking certain drugs, or pregnant, you are at an increased risk. Keep in mind that some minerals compete for absorption, so taking a large dose of one mineral may deplete your body's absorption of another mineral.

DAILY OPTIMAL VITAMIN AND MINERAL SUPPLEMENTATION

The following recommendations for daily intake levels of vitamins and minerals are designed to provide an optimum intake range for maintaining good health. If possible, buy natural, organic vitamins, preferably labeled as not having sugar, preservatives, lactose, yeast, or starch. Also follow instructions regarding storage and recommended dosage. Some minerals and vitamins are toxic in high doses, and the safe dose can be exceeded if you take supplements from more than one source.

VITAMINS	SUPPLEMENTARY DOSAGE RANGE
Vitamin A (retinal)	5,000-10,000 IU
Vitamin A (from beta-carotene)	10,000-75,000 IU
Vitamin D	100-400 IU
Vitamin E (d-alpha tocopherol)	400-1,200 IU
Vitamin K (phytonadione)	60-900 mcg
Vitamin C (ascorbic acid)	500-9,000 mg
Vitamin B1 (thiamine)	10-90 mg
Vitamin B2 (riboflavin)	10-90 mg
Niacin	10-90 mg
Niacin amide	10-30 mg
Vitamin B6 (pyridoxine)	25-100 mg
Biotin	100-300 mcg
Pantothenic acid	25-100 mg

Folic acid	400-1,000 mcg
Vitamin B12	400-1,000 mcg
Choline	150-500 mg
Inositol	150-500 mg

Super Minerals

Minerals are nutrients that function alongside of vitamins as components of body enzymes. While they are needed in small amounts, they are absolutely essential for the biochemical processes of the body to work. Without your minerals in adequate supply, you can't absorb the vitamins.

MINERALS	SUPPLEMENTARY DOSAGE RANGE
Boton	1-2 mg
Calcium	250-750 mg
Chromium	200-400 mcg
Copper	1-2 mg
Iodine	50-150 mcg
Iron	15-30 mg
Magnesium	250-750 mg
Manganese (citrate)	10-15 mg
Molybdenum (sodium molybdate)	10-25 mcg
Potassium	200-500 mg
Selenium (selenomethionine)	100-200 mcg
Silica (sodium metasilicate)	200-1,000 mcg
Vanadium (sulfate)	50-100 mcg
Zinc (picolinate)	15-30 mg

QUESTIONS & ANSWERS

1. Do I have to fast to detoxify?

While there are various methods of detoxifying, fasting is the most effective. Just by eliminating sugars and processed chemically laden foods, you will instantly begin to feel the effects of detoxifying or ridding your body of toxins. Isaiah 58:8 says that by fasting your health will quickly appear.

2. Will I have to give up coffee to be healthy?

Moderation is always the key. However, if you are in bondage to anything, including coffee, you have a problem. God does not want us to be in bondage to anything. He wants us free. Coffee is a poison to your system and should not be taken on a frequent basis. If you are in a state of disease, you should not drink coffee. But an occasional cup of java is okay for a well person.

3. I can't seem to lose weight. What should I do?

First, you need to discern the root of the problem. It could be related to your thyroid, liver, overeating, a sedentary lifestyle, *Candida Albicans*, prescription drug side effects, food addictions, wrong food choices, or something else. The key is to understand why you are where you are and then take action. Don't expect that because a weight-loss program worked for a friend it will work for you. Deal with your specific situation and set realistic goals. Keep in mind that you didn't gain the weight overnight, and it won't come off overnight. Be patient, pray, and don't forget to thank God when the answer comes. Read the chapters on fasting and the Levitical diet, exercise, drinking the recommended water, and consider adding bladder wrack to your diet.

4. I've already detoxified. Do I have to do it again?

Do you only clean your house once? No, you clean it on a regular basis and also do special projects—painting, carpet cleaning, washing windows, etc. And your body is a temple of God (1 Corinthians 6:19)! All the more reason to clean house (detoxify) on a regular basis. We live in a toxic world, and it is imperative to live a fasted life in order to stay as healthy as possible. I recommend, at the minimum, a juice fast once a month for three consecutive days.

5. I don't sleep well. What can I do?

Do you awake during the hours of 2 and 3 A.M.? That is when the liver is at its peak of activity, followed by the pancreas at 3 A.M. If there's a problem with either organ, it's possible you experience low blood sugar and physical and emotional drops by midafternoon. Waking up during this time is usually a signal from your liver to alert you that things aren't quite right. The first step is to cleanse your liver. I'll tell you how to do that in answer to my next question.

You should also check your stress level. It may be that your subconscious is working overtime. Of course, there are many other potential reasons why you may not sleep well, but several natural therapies are readily available at your local health food store that do not involve prescribed drugs (which may have bad side effects). Natures Valerian, which was the predecessor to Valium, is my favorite organic muscle relaxer. Many people benefit from Melatonin, which causes your body to release seritonin and allows you to fall asleep. A liquid or powdered Calcium-Magnesium combination is a magnificent way to induce the deep state of sleep that is really needed by most people. B-complex is also very helpful because B vitamins are what our body uses to fight stress.

6. How can I cleanse my liver?

An excellent way to stimulate the liver to detoxify itself is with coffee enemas. We refer to this as a "Liver Cleanse." They are not for the function of cleansing the intestines. This enema is most often used in metabolic cancer therapy and is extremely valuable in many successful detoxification programs. Coffee enemas alkalinize the first part of the intestines, enhance enzyme function, and stimulate the production and release of bile. The coffee is absorbed through the colon wall and travels via the portal vein directly to the liver. When it stimulates the liver to produce bile, it can cause nausea. A little nausea is desirable, but if it is too great, reduce the amount of coffee used or use the enema on a full stomach. The coffee should be stronger than for drinking. Do no dilute the coffee.

The type of coffee to be used is ground (drip) coffee, not instant or decaffeinated. Mix 2 tablespoons of coffee to 1 quart of steam-distilled water. Use 2 cups at body temperature, twice daily. Take this enema preferably on your knees or lie down on your back, legs drawn close to abdomen, and breathe deeply while the enema is given slowly. Retain the fluid for 10 to 15 minutes.

To detoxify the liver in serious conditions, take two coffee enemas per day. Follow this routine for two weeks, then coffee enemas should be reduced to only one per week for one month.

Your body may have a buildup of toxins or poisons from time to time. Symptoms indicating toxicity are a decrease in appetite, headaches, increase in tiredness, and a general lack of well-being. When these occur, increase coffee enemas once again to one per day until symptoms subside or for a maximum of three to four days.

I also recommend a liver dysfunction diet, which is designed to bring healing to the liver. It must contain high-quality protein, such as white turkey meat, leg of lamb, wild game, white low-fat cheese, yogurt, cottage cheese, goat's milk, sprouted seeds and grains, raw nuts (especially almonds), and sesame butter or ground sesame seeds sprinkled over food, raw and steamed vegetables of all kinds.

Small, frequent meals are preferred rather than two or three large ones. Raw, fresh vegetables and fruits, free of artificial colors, preservatives, or chemicals of any kind, are a must. Avoid all animal fats, canned and refined foods, synthetic vitamins, drugs, strong spices, sugar, coffee, black tea, and alcohol.

The best juices at this time are carrot/celery/parsley with one teaspoon of cream for every eight ounces of juice, red beet (excellent), cucumber, papaya, blue grapes, lemon, and green juice. The best herbs are dandelion, St. John's Wort, lobelia, parsley, horsetail, birch leaves, and sarsaparilla. The best herb teas are peppermint, spearmint, chamomile, thyme, milk thistle, and licorice.

7. Can I get rid of arthritis?

God made our bodies to heal! Detox, detox, detox. I can't say it enough when it comes to arthritis. Your diet has a great influence on joint pain. Stay away from nightshade vegetables such as tomatoes, turnip greens, etc.—they're a major culprit! Go for fresh, uncooked, organic fruits and vegetables low in sugar, and only use sea salt. Try MSM, Glucosamine Sulfate, and Shark Cartledge. Most important of all, drink plenty of steam-distilled water, using the half an ounce per pound method—if you weigh 100 pounds, you would drink 50 ounces of water, which is a little less than 2 quarts per day.

8. I don't have a juicer. Can I still fast?

Yes, start where you are! Almost everyone has a blender, and there are terrific shakes you can get that really work. My favorite is *Creation's Bounty*, which is full of greens, antioxidants, vitamins, minerals, etc. This way you're still ingesting only top quality liquids without the expense of a juicer. Remember that there are juice bars in some health food stores as well as businesses that specialize in juices. Try to use only organic juices if at all possible. Depending on what it is you're trying to accomplish (weight loss, detoxifying, spiritual enrichment, disease related), there's a fast for you, whether it is vegetable, fruit, water, etc. A tailor-made scientific fast designed by our labs could be ordered if you require a fast of 20 days or longer.

9. Do I take my vitamins while fasting?

Only if they are food based. During a fast, it's best to leave off the pills you don't have to take. The less your body has to break down, the more it has time to work on the healing process. However, you should not stop taking any medication unless your doctor says it's okay.

10. How long should I fast?

First, you need to know that juice fasting is the most effective way to restore your health back to the way God intended. Typically, the best place to start is from one to three days. Then after checking with your physician, you may want to go for a longer fast. Everyone is different, but a good rule of thumb is that by fasting three days a month you can extend your life five to seven years. I have individual protocols that can last up to 40 days but require an assessment and dialogue of your current condition before one can be tailor-made for you. Always remember to check with your doctor before starting an extended fasting program.

11. How can I improve my immune system?

Here are the basics you must do to build your immune

system. These can be tweaked for your special needs.

■ Detoxify

■ Increase your oxygen levels in every way possible, including using my *Body Oxygen*™ liquid.

■ Drink half your body weight in ounces of water daily.

■ Eat at least five fresh fruits and/or veggies daily.

■ Consume half a cup of oat bran daily.

■ Take Vitamin C and E and CoQ 10 daily.

■ Always keep a clean temple.

12. I'm tired all the time!

Start investigating why you're tired, because you shouldn't be. It might be due to a bad diet, a lack of exercise, anemia, or an emotional problem, but it could be much more serious. It's never a bad idea to get routine blood work done to make sure everything is okay. If you come back with a clean bill of health, that's always reassuring.

13. Do I have to become a vegetarian?

No. While I don't care for red meat, I do eat it occasionally. I believe the Levitical plan is the way to go. It's balanced and written by the Great Physician. That works for me!

14. What kind of vitamins should I take?

Always take a food-based vitamin. Make sure you buy from a health food store that knows the company that manufactures the product you are interested in. Synthetics can be more harmful than good. A food-based vitamin is made from real foods! People often tell me they feel sick when they take vitamins, and I say the pill must be sick. Change brands and experience the difference.

15. What can I do about depression?

Although there are solid medical reasons why some people experience depression, the percentage is very small in comparison to the depression that is caused by a poor diet. In regions of the world where proper amounts of essential fatty acids (Omega 3, 6, and 9) are consumed through a diet high in fish, depression is unheard of! Less than 1 percent of the people in these cultures ever experience depression. Start with an EFA, cut out salt, sugar, and junk food, and go from there.

16. Is there anything I can do to get my sex drive back?

A few years ago I received a call from a woman who was at the point of desperation. She was about thirty years old, had two young children, and was happily married. Everything in her life seemed to be going well except for this one problem: she had no desire for sex. She loved her husband but physically had no desire to become intimate with him. Her doctor had recommended she see a counselor, who had determined that there must be something deep in her subconscious that was holding her back.

She called because she was too embarrassed to ask me in person whether I thought the counselor was correct. I told her that I really thought her hormones might out of balance because she had a child around three years old. She was so desperate to please her husband that she rushed to my office almost before I could get off the phone. I simply recommended an herbal combination to stimulate the female hormones. The result was perhaps the most elated client and client's spouse I've ever had! She called a few weeks later and said her husband was a happy, happy man, and he had told her she could come see me anytime she wanted.

So what was that herbal combination? Well, have you ever heard of sowing your oats? This is it! The herb is called Avena Sativa, and its common name is Green Oats. Another one that really works is called Horny Goat Weed. These are herbs that naturally stimulate the sexual hormones. There are different combinations for men and women. Yohimbe, Guarana, Taurine, Arginine, and Ornithine are amino acids associated with arousal, erection, and stamina. Remember, God intended for us to enjoy intimacy with our spouse. If one or both of you are unfulfilled, don't think it has to stay that way.

Other reasons for a lack of sex drive can be due to side effects from prescription drugs, disease in the body, or hypothyroidism (an underactive thyroid). Hypothyroidism has become a huge problem in the United States. I have heard the numbers are as high as 1 out of 4 Americans suffer from this disorder. If you have it, take extra care of your liver. The thyroid is responsible for your sex drive, and if your thyroid is low, so goes your sex drive. Happy thyroid = Happy sex drive!

17. I can't have a bowel movement without a laxative or a cup of coffee. What should I do?

I'll just be blunt with this one! I think bowel movements are so important that even my six-year-old knows that if someone is in the bathroom too long, they must be constipated! This subject is rarely talked about in most households and seldom taken as seriously as it should be. Constipation can lead to health problems and even disease of the bowels if not taken care of properly.

If you're eating three meals a day, you should have at least two bowel movements a day. If you're not, consider the food you're eating. Pizza dough, for instance, takes up to three days to pass through your bowels. Just think of that dough turning into cement in your colon the next time you order your double pepperoni!

So, #1—Don't eat things you know are going to back you up. #2—Do eat a half cup of oat bran every day. #3—Take a good pro-biotic to put the good bacteria back into your colon, and it will help you break down the food you take in and eliminate it from your system quicker. #4—Don't be afraid to use a good colon cleanse. Be sure to get one that's recommended by a health care professional (just because it's on the shelf somewhere doesn't mean it's good for you). #5—Consider a colonic on an occasional basis to get into those hard to reach areas in the intestines that have been backed up for years. (Beware! You will be shocked at what comes out.)

18. Is there anything I can do to help prevent cancer?

First, you need to stand on the Word of God and believe that "by his [Christ's] wounds we are healed" (Isaiah 53:5). Nevertheless, faith without works is dead, so you have to do your part to guard against the toxic environment that you're living in too. While there are many things that can be done, here are a few of the basics.

The most important step is to drink half your body weight in ounces of steam distilled water daily. For example, if you weigh 128 pounds, you should drink 2 quarts or 4 pints of water every day, but not all at once. Start your morning with a glass, then continue throughout the day. This will help to flush out the toxins and a wide variety of other waste products.

According to the American Cancer Society, by eating five fresh fruits and vegetables every day you can cut your risk of cancer by 30 percent. But if you cook the vegetables, they don't count. Vegetables need to be raw or lightly steamed. Also, by eating one half cup of oat bran daily you can cut your risk of cancer another 30 percent. I like *All Bran®* cereal.

One more essential regarding cancer is selenium. If you have had cancer, you might want to consume 600 mg of selenium per day. If cancer runs in your family, consider 400 mg daily. And just as a preventative measure, a healthy person might take 200 mg daily. By taking this very inexpensive trace mineral, which used to be found abundantly in our natural foods, studies show that you can cut your risk of cancer another 50 percent! Wow!

Another important step is to increase your oxygen levels. Perform deep breathing exercises, use the Chi machine, go for walks, supplement with Silver Creeks' *Body Oxygen™*, and consider antioxidants to stop free radical damage. Start with these simple steps and work your way up.

19. What can I do about high cholesterol?

Change your eating habits! Most people's problem is what they're putting in their mouths. We tend to think that cholesterol is handed down genetically. I believe it has more to do with recipes passed down from Grandma, and thus the same disorders are passed down. If you do not deal with your diet, all the other helps in the world won't make a difference.

You also need to consider the natural products that God has given us to lower bad cholesterol levels. According to the American Cholesterol Foundation, niacin (vitamin B-3) brings bad cholesterol levels down as much or more than the leading prescription drugs. Niacin costs pennies per day and can easily be found at your local health food store. Some people complain about the niacin flush, which may feel prickly for up to a half hour, but they need to realize that is the only side effect. Niacin does not threaten to do liver damage, unlike the cholesterol drugs that are being prescribed by most physicians. The added benefit of a niacin flush is that your skin pushes out toxins and increases oxygen flow to the surface, and thus you have a more youthful look!

Another natural product that works well to lower bad cholesterol is Red Yeast Rice. It has developed a great following.

20. What can be done to naturally bring down high blood pressure?

Many studies have shown that *Olive Leaf Extract*™ brings down high blood pressure in all mammals. Garlic also works great. I like *Kyolic®*, which is odor free and found in any health food store. The benefits are endless!

Once again, your diet is the key to bringing down high blood pressure. If you think a high fat diet isn't a factor, you're dreaming. In extreme cases I highly recommend chelation therapies. This cleans the plaque from the arteries, thus bringing the blood pressure down while performing a number of other health services for the patient. A complete list of medical doctors who are trained in Chelation and other complementary treatments are listed in the back of this book.

21. What can I do about PMS and menopause?

Women and men both love the answer to this question. Women love it because they suffer from it, and men because they have to deal with it. But it can be helped, and in a big way. I truly thank God that I haven't had to deal with PMS for the majority of my adult life because I've been very cautious to not put harmful chemicals into my body that greatly affect the hormone balances in the body (such as birth control pills or milk filled with bovine hormones).

The answer is to take 1,200-1,500 mg of Evening Primrose Oil and 200–400 IUs of Vitamin E twice a day. Increase the Vitamin E up to 1,000 IUs daily until night sweats and symptoms decrease. This is so easy. It also gives you essential fatty acids, aids your brain functions, helps your skin and joints, and much more.

This simple combination works so well that my own teenage daughters have been known on occasion to have their teachers call me to get this little remedy. The teachers love it and pass it on to their colleagues, and my daughters score a few extra points with the teachers. I use this advice myself! I really like the way it affects me in a number of ways, especially my curly hair.

Give it a try for 30–60 days, and you'll love it! It's simple, inexpensive, and has only good side effects. Add a good food-based B complex to it, and you soon will be another one of my great testimonials.

22. Does anything work on acne and skin conditions?

I know I sound like a broken record, but I have to say it again. What's on the inside will come out. If you are toxic, it will show! If you have acne, psoriasis, eczema, or other skin problems, you must clean your insides. It won't work to just paint the outside. Drink water, fast, and detoxify, then follow the diet I've outlined in this book. You may discover that even your liver spots disappear.

Second, make sure you are using natural skin products. Chemicals can be the source of reactions on your skin.

Third, make sure you are getting your required essential fatty acids. These are ever so important for beautiful skin.

23. I am stressed all the time. Is there anything I can do?

First of all, no matter what is happening in your life, cast your cares upon the Lord, for He cares for you. "Come to me," Jesus said, "all you who are weary and burdened, and I will give you rest. Take my yoke upon you and learn from me, for I am gentle and humble in heart, and you will find rest for your souls. For my yoke is easy and my burden is light" (Matthew 11:28-30). Always bring Jesus alongside of your life and receive His rest, and if the stress points in your situation can be changed, do it!

Keep in mind that when you are stressed out, your minerals and B vitamins can be depleted in one hour. This is why a person so often feels exhausted after receiving bad news or when an additional care is heaped upon other cares. The immune system has also been compromised during stress. Be prepared for these times and keep yourself built up. Take a liquid mineral supplement along with a good food-based B-Complex and folic acid.

If you feel you must have something to relax you, try valerian extract. It's a great herb that really works to help a person unwind. And eat or drink lots of celery, which some call nature's Valium.

24. I have constant back pain. What can I take other than drugs with all the side effects?

If you are overweight and have a large belly that pulls on the back, you can expect to have back pain. First, you have to lose the weight, and then you need to exercise to the level where your abdominal muscles can support your spine and keep it exactly where it should be.

Second, ask your friends and acquaintances if they know a good chiropractor. A good chiropractor can be worth his or her weight in gold!

Consider asking your doctor about Glucosamine Sulfate, which according to German studies is absorbed much easier than the Glucosamine Condrotin. There are also several combinations that have MSM in them. The sulfur in the MSM can do wonders for many ailments.

The most recent products are the ones with a Cox2 enzyme inhibitor. These work by actually blocking the very thing that causes the pain and inflammation. The Cox2 enzyme is also associated with other dis-eases such as heart disease!

25. I eat really well and take lots of supplements. So why am I still sick?

An old doctor once said that there is no disease that cannot be cured, only patients that cannot. I know that sounds harsh, but the more people I counsel, the more I realize that a good attitude and a forgiven and clean heart have so much to do with healing. We usually think of toxins as something that comes in from the outside. But with toxic thinking, we can produce toxins on our own. No amount of cleansing and detoxifying will remove bitterness, unforgiveness, fear, or any other bad attitude that shouldn't be there.

Ask our wonderful heavenly Father for wisdom so that you can pluck out the real root and be free and healthy all the time.

26. Can anything be done for Fibromyalgia Syndrome?

There are many other things that can be done, but this is where you start. Anything that helps to oxygenate your body, such as a daily dose of 75 mg of Coenzyme Q-10. *Body Oxygen*™ and *Clustered Water*™ can make a real difference. *Candida* infections are common in people with fibromyalgia, so hit it hard with a good pro-biotic. I like Natren's Trenev Trio. I have not seen a pro-biotic even close to its quality. A good liquid calcium magnesium is excellent right before bed.

27. What about Chronic Fatigue?

By simply detoxifying, you may see the difference between night and day. A good Vitamin C flush is inexpensive and easy. Go to your local health food store and get crystalized Vitamin C. Mix 25,000 mg of Vitamin C with your favorite non-sugary juice. You may need to split this up into several servings. Be warned: you will have a lot of diarrhea! What this is doing is taking you to bowel tolerance. This is a good thing—you will be clean. At the end of the three-day cleansing, start taking Natren's Trenev Trio and continue for 60 days. This has been used by people in various stages of Chronic Fatigue, and I have to say that the results are almost too good to be true.

28. I am suffering from Adult Onset Diabetes or Type II Diabetes. Is there anything I can do?

While this is not a new disorder, the number of people diagnosed with it in recent years is alarming. However, it is amazing that AOD is basically unheard of in third world countries. Some people have nicknamed AOD "The Prosperity Disease," because the causes of AOD are not available in impoverished nations.

An interesting fact is that while AOD has been studied for years, the rise in numbers did not come until 1988.

This was the year that Aspartame was introduced into the American diet. Each year the average American consumes 148 pounds of artificial sweeteners. Our bodies are simply not made to process chemicals, including this one. The troubling fact is someone with AOD reaches for artificial sweetener because they're told to not take in sugars.

I personally believe that Type II Diabetes is reversible for most people. The key is you. You must stop the habits that got you there to begin with. All of these are contributing factors to AOD—processed foods, artificial sweeteners, a sedentary lifestyle, and bad fats such as hydrogenated oils. Also, you need to stay away from extreme plans such as high protein diets or high carb diets. God set forth a plan in the Levitical diet (see chapter 9), which brings a balance in protein, carbohydrates, and good fats and doesn't include insulin resistance.

If you are overweight, you need to lose the extra pounds as soon as possible! Start an exercise program, and select one that you will keep up with. You also need to detoxify your body and give your liver a chance to start assimilating the nutrients you take in. Get on a good regimen of nutritional supplements. Oxygen helps every bodily function, so practice deep breathing exercises daily. Try Chromium GTF (the "GTF" means glucose tolerance factors). Vitamin E, Lipoic Acid, B-complex, a liquid mineral supplement, and a good food-based multivitamin are essential for health and recovery.

APPENDIX A

AMERICA'S LEADING COMPLEMENTARY ALTERNATIVE MEDICAL DOCTORS

THE ACAM (AMERICAN COLLEGE FOR ADVANCE-MENT IN MEDICINE) is a medical society devoted to the education of medical professionals. The following list of more than 775 of America's leading complimentary alternative medical doctors is information provided on its Web site (www.acam.org) and is for educational purposes only. ACAM does not provide medical advice to the public. Please check with a physician if you suspect you are ill or are in need of specific medical advice. ACAM does offer the public two excellent resources: (1) A doctor search, and (2) ACAM book catalog.

LIST OF ABBREVIATIONS

A—allergy
AA—anti-aging
AN—anesthesiology
AC—acupuncture
AR—arthritis
AU—auriculotherapy
BA—bariatrics
CD—cardiovascular disease
CT—chelation therapy
CS—chest disease
DD—degenerative disease
DIA—diabetes
END—endocrinology
FP—family practice
GD—general dentistry
GE—gastroenterology
GP—general practice
GER—geriatrics
GYN—gynecology
HGL—hypoglycemia
HO—hyperbaric oxygen
HOM—homeopathy
HYP—hypnosis
IM—internal medicine
LM—legal medicine
MM—metabolic medicine

NT—nutrition
OBS—obstetrics
OD—orthodontia
OME—orthomolecular
    medicine
ON—oncology
OPH—ophthalmology
OSM—osteopathic
    manipulation
PD—pediatrics
PM—preventive medicine
PMR—physical medicine
    & rehabilitation
P—psychiatry
PO—psychiatry
    (orthomolecular)
PH—public health
P/S—prolotherapy/
    sclerotherapy
PUD—pulmonary diseases
R—radiology
RHU—rheumatology
RHI—rhinology
S—surgery
WR—weight reduction
YS—yeast syndrome

ALABAMA

BIRMINGHAM

Michael S. Vaughn, MD
One Lakeshore Dr., #100
Birmingham, AL 35209
(205) 930-2950
DIA,FP,IM,NT,PM,YS

DAPHNE

Charles Runels Jr., MD
7146 Stone Drive
Daphne, AL 36526
(334) 625-2612
FAX (334) 625-2615
BA,CT,DIA,PMR,IM,CD

Glen P. Wilcoxson, MD
P.O. Box 1347
Daphne, AL 36526
(334) 447-0333
FAX (334) 447-0009
BA,CT,NT,PM,RHU,YS

FOLEY

Edward D. Hubbard, MD
224 Laurel Ave. West
Foley, AL 36535
(334) 943-9430
CT,DD,GP,HYP,P/S

GULF SHORES

Gregory S. Funk, DO, BPCT
2103 W. 1st Street
P.O. Box 2029
Gulf Shores, AL 36547
(334) 968-2441
FAX (334) 968-5555
FP,GP,OS

HEFLIN

Gus J. Prosch Jr., MD
P.O. Box 427
Helflin, AL 36264
(205) 222-0960
FAX (256) 748-3126
Email: gusd@hiwaay.net
A,AR,CT,GP,NT,OME

MONTGOMERY

Teresa D. Allen, DO, APCT
6715 Taylor Court
Montgomery, AL 36117
(334) 273-0904
FAX (334) 273-0905
CT,IM,NT,OS,PM,P/S

Scott Bell, MD
7020 Sydney Curve
Montgomery, AL 36117
(334) 277-5363
FAX (334) 277-5362
Email: scottabell@dnamail.com
PM,IM,CT,AA

ALASKA

ANCHORAGE

Sandra Denton, MD, APCT
3201 C Street, Suite 602
Anchorage, AK 99503
(907) 563-6200
FAX (907) 561-4933
Email: aamc@myexcel.com
A,AC,AR,AU,CD,CT,DD,DIA,END,
FP,NT

Robert Rowen, MD, APCT
615 E. 82nd Ave., Suite 300
Anchorage, AK 99518
(907) 344-7775
FAX (907) 522-3114
AC,CT,FP,HYP,NT,PM,P/S

Robert Thompson, MD
3333 Denali Street, #100
Anchorage, AK 99503
(907) 563-6200
FAX (907) 561-4933
OB-GYN

PALMER

D. Lynn Mickleson, MD, BPCT
440-A West Evergreen
Palmer, AK 99645
(907) 745-3880
FAX (907) 745-2631
A,CT,GP

SOLDOTNA

Elisabeth-Anne Cole, MD, APCT
43335 K-Beach Road #8
Soldotna, AK 99669
(907) 262-7977
FAX (907) 262-9174

WASILLA

Robert E. Martin, MD
P.O. Box 870710
Wasilla, AK 99687
(907) 376-5284
Email: rmartin@micronet.net
AU,CT,FP,GP,OS,PM,P/S

ARIZONA

APACHE JUNCTION

David Korn, DO, MD (H)
11518 E. Apache Trail, #115
Apache Junction, AZ 85220
(480) 354-6700
FAX (480) 354-6708

CASA GRANDE

Charles D. Schwengel, DO, MD (H)
1927 N. Trekell Rd., #A
Casa Grande, AZ 85222
(520) 836-7441
CT,HOM,NT,OME,PM

CAVE CREEK

Frank W. George, DO, MD (H), BPCT
6748 E. Lone Mountain Rd.
Cave Creek, AZ 85254
(480) 595-5508
FAX (480) 575-1570
Email: fwg336@pol.net
CT,DD,GP,MM,NT,OS

FLAGSTAFF

Marnie Vail, MD
702 North Beaver Street
Flagstaff, AZ 86001
(928) 214-9774
FAX (928) 214-9772
Email: marnie@safeaccess.com
FP,HOM,CT

GANADO

Clifford B. Bell, MD
Sage Memorial Hospital
Ganado, AZ 86505
(520) 755-3411, Ext. 310
Aviation Med., OPH

GLENDALE

Lloyd D. Arnold, DO, MD (H), APCT
4901 W. Bell Rd., Suite 2
Glendale, AZ 85308
(602) 939-8916
FAX (602) 978-2817
Email: Doc_Armold@bigfoot.com
AR,CT,GP,MM,PM,OSM

MESA

Thomas J. Grade, MD
6641 E. Baywood, #A-2
Mesa, AZ 85206
(480) 981-2992
FAX (480) 981-1309
AC,AN,AU,CT,IM,PUD

William W. Halcomb, MD (H)
4323 E. Broadway, Suite 109
Mesa, AZ 85206
(602) 832-3014
FAX (602) 832-5216
A,CT,GP,HO,OSM,PM

Charles D. Schwengel, DO, MD (H)
1050 E. University, #4
Mesa, AZ 85203
(602) 668-1448
CT,HOM,NT,OME,OSM,PM

PARKER

Jeff A. Baird, DO, BPCT
1413 – 16th Street
Parker, AZ 85344
(520) 669-9229
AC,CT,FP,OS

PAYSON

Garry F. Gordon, MD, DO, MD (H), APCT
708 E. Hwy., 260, Bldg. C-1, #F
Payson, AZ 85541
(520) 472-4263
FAX (520) 474-3819
Email: drgary@netzone.com

PHOENIX

Gary G. Bucher, MD
4455 E. Camelback Rd., #B-100
Phoenix, AZ 85018
(602) 667-0007
FAX (602) 778-1998
FP

Alan K. Ketover, MD, MD (H)
10565 N. Tatum Blvd., #B-115
Phoenix, AZ 85253
(602) 381-0800
A,CT,HOM,NT,PM,YS,Env. Med.

Edward C. Kondrot, MD, BPCT
5501 N. 19th Avenue
Phoenix, AZ 85015
(602) 347-7950
CT,NT,HOM

Stanley R. Olsztyn, MD (H)
Suite B-220
4350 E. Camelback Rd.
Phoenix, AZ 85018
(602) 840-8424
FAX (602) 840-8545
A,CT,PM,DD

Geoffrey Radoff, MD (H)
2525 W. Greenway Rd., #210
Phoenix, AZ 85018
(602) 993-0200
FAX (602) 993-0207
FP

Bruce H. Shelton, MD (H), BPCT
2525 W. Greenway Rd., #300
Phoenix, AZ 85018
(602) 993-1200
FAX (602) 942-3787
A,AC,DD,FP,HOM,PO,YS

SCOTTSDALE

Gordon H. Josephs, DO, MD (H), APCT
7315 E. Evans Road
Scottsdale, AZ 85260
(480) 998-9232
FAX (480) 998-1528
Email: gjosephs@pol.net
CT,CD,DIA,NT,OME,YS

SEDONA

Lester Adler, MD
40 Soldiers Pass Rd., #12
Sedona, AZ 86336
(520) 282-2520
CT,GP,IM,MM,NT,P/S,PM

Mark E. Laursen, MD
150 Thunderbird Drive
Sedona, AZ 86336
(520) 204-0023
FAX (520) 204-1571
GP,Emerg. Med.

Annemarie S. Welch, MD
2301 West Hwy. 89A, #104
Sedona, AZ 86336
(520) 282-0609
IM,CT,NT,YS,DD,PM

SHOW LOW

William W. Halcomb, MD (H)
2000 N. 16th Ave.
Show Low, AZ 85901
(602) 832-3014
FAX (602) 832-5216
A,CT,GP,HO,OSM,PM

SUN CITY

Frank W. George, DO, MD (H), BPCT
12611 No. 103rd Ave., #A
Sun City, AZ 85351
(623) 876-9045
FAX (623) 876-8854
Email: fwg336@pol.net
CT,DD,GP,MM,NT,OS

TUCSON

Alexander P. Cadoux, MD (H), APCT
6884 E. Sunrise Dr., #150
Tucson, AZ 85750-0829
(520) 529-9668
FAX (520) 529-9669
A,CT,FP,MM,NT,PM

Woody McGinnis, MD
3150 Cerrada Los Palitos
Tucson, AZ 85718
NO REFERRALS

Jesse Stoff, MD (H), APCT
3402 East Broadway
Tucson, AZ 85716
(520) 319-9074
FAX (520) 319-9073
A,AC,CT

ARKANSAS

LITTLE ROCK

Norbert J. Becquet, MD, FACAM, APCT
613 Main Street
Little Rock, AR 72201
(501) 375-4419
FAX (501) 375-4067
AR,CT,OPH,PM,RHU,Pain Control

MOUNTAIN HOME

Merl B. Cox, DO
1613 Hwy. 62 E
Mountain Home, AR 72653
(870) 424-5025
FAX (870) 425-3922
OS,PM,CT

SPRINGDALE

Jeffrey R. Baker, MD
900 Dorman St., #E
Springdale, AR 72762
(501) 756-3251
CT,FP,NT,PM,YS,GP

CALIFORNIA

ATASCADERO

Carmelo A. Plateroti, DO, BPCT
8548 El Camino Real
Atascadero, CA 93422
(805) 462-2262
FAX (805) 462-2264
CT,DD,END,NR,PM, Dermatology

AZUSA

William C. Bryce, MD
400 N. San Gabriel Ave.
Azusa, CA 91702-3446
(626) 334-1407
FAX (626) 334-1116
CT,NT,PM

BEVERLY HILLS

Cathie Ann Lippman, MD
291 S. La Cienega Bl., Suite 207
Beverly Hills, CA 90211
(310) 289-8430
A,AC,PM,YS

Barry Solof, MD
8306 Wilshire Blvd., #311
Beverly Hills, CA 90211
(323) 874-9947
FAX (323) 850-1415
IM,GER,FP,Addiction Medicine

BURBANK

David J. Edwards, MD
2202 W. Magnolia
Burbank, CA 91506
(818) 842-4184
(800) 975-2202
A,AR,CD,CT,NT,OME,RHU,WR,YS

Douglas Hunt, MD
3808 Riverside Dr., #510
Burbank, CA 91505
(818) 566-9889
FAX (818) 566-9879
A,BA,CT, HGL,MM,NT,PM,PO,YS

Nancy T. Mullan, MD
2829 West Burbank Blvd., #202
Burbank, CA 91505
(818) 954-9267
FAX (818) 954-0620
P,PO,YS,Child PO,GYN,
Menopause

Sion Nobel, MD
1130 W. Olive Ave., #B
Burbank, CA 91506
(818) 845-0505
FAX (818) 361-9497
Email: snobelmd@aol.com
CT,PM,PMR,P/S,Pain Mgmt.

BURNEY

Charles K. Dahlgren, MD
37491 Enterprise Dr., #C
Burney, CA 96013
(530) 335-3833
A,NT,RHI,S

CARMEL

Gerald A. Wyker, MD
25530 Rio Vista Drive
Carmel, CA 93923
(831) 625-0911
FAX (831) 625-0467
Email: jerry@wyker-md.com
CT,Long./Anti-Aging, NT,PM

CARMICHAEL

Bernard McGinity, MD
6945 Fair Oaks Blvd.
Carmichael, CA 95608
(916) 485-4556
FAX (916) 485-1491
GP,AC,HYP,NT,YS

Philip J Reilly, MD
4800 Manzanita Ave., #17
Carmichael, CA 95608
(916) 488-9524
AU,FP,P/S

CHULA VISTA

Luis Perez, MD
790 Otay Lakes Rd.
Chula Vista, CA 91910
(619) 216-1600
FAX (619) 216-1616
DIA,GP,PM,P/S,R

COLTON

Bruce W. Halstead, MD
23000 Grand Terrace Rd.
Colton, CA 92324
HONORARY MEMBER

CONCORD

John Toth, DO
2299 Bacon St., #11
Concord, CA 94520
(510) 687-9447
FAX (510) 687-9483
A,CT,FP,NT,PMR

John P. Toth, MD, APCT
2299 Bacon St., Suite 10
Concord, CA 94520
(925) 682-5660
FAX (925) 682-8097
A,CD,CT,GP,HGL,NT

COVINA

James Privitera, MD
105 No. Grandview Ave.
Covina, CA 91723
(626) 966-1618
FAX (626) 966-7226
A,CT,MM,NT

EL CAJON

Neil W. Hirschenbein, MD
1685 E. Main St., #301
El Cajon, CA 92021
(619) 579-8681
FAX (619) 579-0759
IM,GE

David A. Howe, MD, BPCT
505 N. Mollison Ave., #103
El Cajon, CA 92021
(619) 440-3838
FAX (760) 489-2238
CT,GP,NT,PM,PMR,P/S

William J. Saccoman, MD, APCT
505 N. Mollison Ave., Suite 103
El Cajon, CA 92021
(619) 440-3838
FAX (619) 440-8293
CT,NT,PM

ENCINITAS

Mark Drucker, MD
4403 Manchester Ave., #107
Encinitas, CA 92024
(760) 632-9042
FAX (760) 632-0574
BA,CT,NT,PM,WR

ENCINO

Ilona Abraham, MD
17815 Ventura Blvd.,
Stes. 111 & 113
Encino, CA 91316
(818) 345-8721
FAX (818) 345-7150
info@antiaging-techniques.com
A,AC,CD,CT,P,Natural Horm.

Priscilla A. Slagle, MD
16550 Ventura Blvd., #405
Encino, CA 91436
(310) 826-0175
FAX (760) 323-4259
A,HYP,NT,PM,PO,YS

ESCONDIDO

Ratibor Pantovich, DO
560 E. Valley Pkwy.
Escondido, CA 92025
(760) 480-2880
FAX (760) 480-0102
BA,CT,OS

FOSTER CITY

Bruce Wapen, MD
985 East Hillsdale Blvd., #278
Foster City, CA 94404
(415) 696-4500
FAX (415) 696-4471
Emerg. Med.

FOUNTAIN VALLEY

Allen Green, MD
18153 Brookhurst St.
Fountain Valley, CA 92708
(714) 378-5656
FAX (714) 378-5650
AC,CT,FP,NT,PM

FRESNO

David J. Edwards, MD
360 S. Clovis Ave.
Fresno, CA 93727
(559) 251-5066
FAX (559) 251-5108
A,AR,CD,CT,NT,OME,RHU,WR,YS

Patrick A. Golden, MD, BPCT
1187 E. Herndon, #101
Fresno, CA 93720
(559) 432-0716
FAX (559) 432-4545
CD,IM

GARDENA

Laszlo I. Belenyessy,
MD—RETIRED
14911 West Kingsley Drive
Gardena, CA 90247
NO REFERRALS

GLENDALE

Abraham Maissian, MD, BPCT
1737 W. Glenoaks Blvd.
Glendale, CA 91201
(818) 243-1186
FAX (818) 243-3868
A,CD,CT,DD,FP,IM,PD

HUNTINGTON BEACH

Francis Foo, MD
10188 Adams Ave.
Huntington Beach, CA 92646
(714) 968-3266
FAX (714) 968-6408
FP,S,CT

INDIO

Robert Harmon, MD
41-800 Washington St., #110
Indio, CA 92201-8154
(619) 345-2696
CT,DD,FP,GP,PM,YS

IRVINE

Allan E. Sosin, MD, APCT
16100 Sand Canyon Ave.
Irvine, CA 92618
(949) 753-8889
FAX (949) 753-0410
CT,CD,DIA,GER,IM,NT

Ronald Wempen, MD, BPCT
14795 Jeffrey Rd., Suite 101
Irvine, CA 92618
(949) 551-8751
FAX (949) 551-1272
Email: elaron@earthlink.net
A,AC,MM,NT,PO,YS

LA JOLLA

Charles Moss, MD
8950 Villa La Jolla, #2162
La Jolla, CA 92037
(619) 457-1314
FAX (619) 457-3615
Email: camossmd@aol.com
AC,FP,HGL,MM,NT, YS, Env. Med.

LAFAYETTE

Richard Gracer, MD
895 Moraga Rd., #15
Lafayette, CA 94549
(925) 283-6590
FAX (925) 277-1358
FP,DD,OME,PM,P/S,CT,OSM,WR

LAGUNA HILLS

Peter Muran, MD, BPCT
23521 Paseo de Valencia, #204
Laguna Hills, CA 92653
(888) 315-4777
FAX (714) 430-1443
BA,FP,GER,PM,YS

LANCASTER

Richard P. Huemer, MD
1739 West Avenue J
Lancaster, CA 93534
(661) 945-4502
FAX (661) 945-4841
A,CT,GP,HGL,MM,NT,OME,PM

Mary Kay Michelis, MD
1739 West Avenue J
Lancaster, CA 93534
(661) 945-4502
FAX (661) 947-5527
OPH

LONG BEACH

H. R. Casdorph, MD, PhD,
FACAM, DIPL
1703 Termino Avel, Suite 201
Long Beach, CA 90804
(562) 597-8716
FAX (562) 597-4616
Email: CASDORPH@AOL.COM
CD,CS,CT,DIA,IM,NT

LOS ALTOS

Robert F. Cathcart III, MD
127 Second St., Suite 4
Los Altos, CA 94022
(650) 949-2822
A,AR,CT,DD,OME,PM

F. T. Guilford, MD
5050 El Camino Real, #110
Los Altos, CA 94022
(650) 964-6700
FAX (650) 433-0947
Email: guilford@flash.net
A,CT,NT,PM

Raj Patel, MD
5050 El Camino Real, #110
Los Altos, CA 94022
(650) 964-6700
FAX (650) 964-3495
A,CT,FP,NT,PM,YS

D. Graeme Shaw, MD
5050 El Camino Real, #110
Los Altos, CA 94022
(650) 964-6700
FAX (650) 964-3495
A,CT,IM,NT,PM,YS

LOS ANGELES

Michael Galitzer, MD
12381 Wilshire Blvd., #102
Los Angeles, CA 90025
(310) 820-6042
FAX (310) 207-3342
mikegal@worldnet.att.net
AC,CT,FP,HOM,NT,OME

Hans D. Gruenn, MD, BPCT
2211 Corinth Ave., #204
Los Angeles, CA 90064
(310) 966-9194
FAX (310) 966-9196
AC,CT,GP,NT,PM,PMR,YS

Howard W. Oliver, DO
5260 S. Figueroa, #110
Los Angeles, CA 90037
(323) 235-1605
FAX (323) 235-1694
GP, OSM

Murray Susser, MD, APCT
2211 Corinth Ave., #204
Los Angeles, CA 90064
(310) 966-9194
FAX (310) 966-9196
A,CT,NT,OME

LOS GATOS

Philip Lee Miller, MD
15215 National Ave., #103
Los Gatos, CA 95032
(408) 358-8855
CD,END,NT,PM,Longv. & Anti-
Aging Med.

MALIBU

Jesse Hanley, MD
21566 Rambla Vista
Malibu, CA 90265
(310) 456-7721
FAX (310) 456-9482
AC,FP,HGL,NT,PM,YS

MARIPOSA

Robert J. Casanas, MD
4979 Hwy. 140, P.O. Box 129
Mariposa, CA 95338
(209) 742-6606
FAX (209) 966-4251
doctorfeelgood@sierratel.com
CT,AC,IM,NT,PM,PMR

MISSION HILLS

Sion Nobel, MD
10306 N. Sepulveda Blvd.
Mision Hills, CA 91345
(818) 361-0115
FAX (818) 361-9497
Email: snobelmd@aol.com
CT,PM,PMR,Pain Mgmt.,Horm.
Repl.

MODESTO

Christine G. Tazewell, MD
1928 Bur Oak Drive
Modesto, CA 95354
NO REFERRALS

MONTEREY

David Anzaldua, MD
172 El Dorado Street
Monterey, CA 93940
(831) 373-1551
Email: intemed1@aol.com
FP

Howard Press, MD
172 El Dorado Street
Monterey, CA 93940
(831) 373-1551
FAX (831) 373-1140
CT,DD,FP,NT,PM,YS

NAPA

Eleanor Hynote, MD
935 Trancas Street, Suite 1A
Napa, CA 94558
(707) 255-4172
FAX (707) 255-2605
AC,CD,IM,NT

NEWPORT BEACH

Julian Whitaker, MD, APCT
4321 Birch St., Suite 100
Newport Beach, CA 92660
(949) 851-1550
FAX (949) 955-3005
CD,CT,DIA,DD,NT,PM

NORTH HOLLYWOOD

Christine Daniel, MD
12650 Sherman Way, #4
North Hollywood, CA 91605
(818) 982-8062
FAX (818) 982-8794
CT,DD,GP,HO,PM,PMR

OAKLAND

Catherine Fehrmann, MD
2424 Stockbridge Dr.
Oakland, CA 94611
NO REFERRALS

OCEANSIDE

Ratibor Pantovich, DO
1002 South Coast Hwy.
Oceanside, CA 92054
(760) 439-9933
FAX (760) 439-3463
BA,CT,OS

ORANGE

James Vatcher, MD, BPCT
872 Cedarwood Street
Orange, CA 92869
NO REFERRALS

PALM DESERT

Robert Neal Rouzier, MD
77564B Country Club Dr., #320
Palm Desert, CA 92211
(760) 772-8883
CT,CD,FP,IM,NT,PM, Natural
Hormones

PALM SPRINGS

Robert Neal Rouzier, MD
2825 Tahquitz Canyon, Suite 200
Palm Springs, CA 92262
(760) 320-4292
FAX (760) 322-9475
CT,CD,FP,IM,NT,PM, Hyperbaric
Med.

Priscilla A. Slagle, MD
946 Avenida Palos Verdes
Palm Springs, CA 92262
(760) 323-4259
FAX (760) 323-4259
A,HYP,NT,PM,PO,YS

RANCHO CUCAMONGA

Francis V. Pau, MD, MD (H)
9726 Foothill Blvd.
Rancho Cucamonga, CA 91730
(909) 987-4262
FAX (909) 987-9542
francispaumdmdh@aol.com
BA,CT,DIA,GP,HOM, IM,NT,P/S

RANCHO MIRAGE

David H. Tang, MD
20 Bentley Road
Rancho Mirage, CA 92270
NO REFERRALS

REDDING

Bessie J. Tillman, MD, APCT
2787 Eureka Way, Suite 1-1
Redding, CA 96001
(530) 246-3022
FAX (530) 246-7894
A,CT,DD,NT,PM,YS

REDLANDS

Felix Prakasam, MD
2048 Orange Tree Lane
Redlands, CA 92374
(909) 798-1614
AN,CT,DD,HO,NT, OSM

SACRAMENTO

Michael Kwiker, DO
3301 Alta Arden, Suite 3
Sacramento, CA 95825
(916) 489-4400
FAX (916) 489-1710
A,CT,DIA,NT

Giovanni Morino, DO
3301 Alta Arden, #3
Sacramento, CA 95825
(916) 489-4400
FAX (916) 489-1710
CT,CD,DIA,FP,NT,OS

SAN DIEGO

Hector R. Fernandez, MD, BPCT
2555 Camino del Rio South,
Suite 207
San Diego, CA 92108
(619) 543-9410
FAX (619) 543-0814
AN

Aline Fournier, DO
307 S. Ivy
Escondido, CA 92025
(760) 746-1133
FAX (760) 746-9880
CT,FP,OS,PM,P/S/YS

Michael I. Leeman, MD
8950 Villa La Jolla Dr., #1162
San Diego, CA 92037
(858) 550-1999
FAX (858) 550-1955
www.longevityclinic.com
CT,CD,END,NT,HO,PM

Romeo A. Quini, MD
458 – 26th Street
San Diego, CA 92102
(619) 234-7398
FAX (760) 839-0299
Email: raq1932@pol.net
AC,CS,CT,FP,GP,PM

SAN FRANCISCO

Catherine Arvantely, MD
345 West Portal Ave.
San Francisco, CA 94127
(415) 566-1000
FAX (415) 665-6732
Email: delphidoc@hotmail.com
FP,NT,PM,CT,OME,GYN

Laurens N. Garlington, MD
56 Scenic Way
San Francisco, CA 94121
NO REFERRALS

Paul Lynn, MD, APCT
345 W. Portal Ave., 2nd Floor
San Francisco, CA 94127
(415) 566-1000
FAX (415) 665-6732
Email: plsfpmg@aol.com
A,AR,CT,DIA,DD,NT,PM,Nat.
Hormones

Wai-Man Ma, MD, BPCT
728 Pacific Ave., #611
San Francisco, CA 94133
(415) 397-3888
FP

Gary Ross, MD
500 Sutter, #300
San Francisco, CA 94102
(415) 398-0555
FAX (415) 398-6228
A,AC,CT,DD,FP,NT,PM

Norman Zucker, MD
711 Van Ness, #330
San Francisco, CA 94102
(800) 799-2250
A,CT,DD,NT,MM,YS

SAN JACINTO

Hiten Shah, MD
229 West 7th
San Jacinto, CA 92583
(909) 487-2550
FAX (909) 487-2552
GP,NT,PM

SAN JOSE

Carl L. Ebnother, MD
7174 Santa Teresa Blvd., #6-A
San Jose, CA 95139
(408) 363-1498
CD,CT,IM,MM,NT,YS

SAN LEANDRO

Steven H. Gee, MD, APCT
595 Estudillo St.
San Leandro, CA 94577
(510) 483-5881
AC,BA,CT,GP

SAN RAMON

Richard Gracer, MD
5401 Norris Canyon Rd., #102
San Ramon, CA 94583
(925) 277-1100
FAX (925) 283-2009
FP,DD,OME,PM,P/S,CT,OSM,WR

SANTA BARBARA

Kenneth J. Frank, MD
831 State St., #280
Santa Barbara, CA 93101
(805) 730-7420
FAX (805) 730-7434
A,BA,FP,NT,PM

James L. Kwako, MD
1805-D East Cabrillo Blvd.
Santa Barbara, CA 93018
(805) 565-3959
FAX (805) 565-3989
AC,CT,FP,NT,PM

Bob Young, MD, BPCT
119 North Milpas
Santa Barbara, CA 93103
(805) 963-1824
FAX (805) 963-1826
CT,CD,DIA,DD,NT,PM,RHU

SANTA MARIA

Nolan T. Higa, MD
615 S. Broadway
Santa Maria, CA 93458
(805) 347-0067/68
FAX (805) 922-2607
AN,CT

SANTA ROSA

Ron Kennedy, MD, APCT
2448 Guerneville Rd., Suite 800
Santa Rosa, CA 95403
(707) 576-0100
Email: nexus@sonic.net
CT,BA,CD,DD,DIA,END,NT

Terri Su, MD
95 Montgomery Dr., #220
Santa Rosa, CA 95404
(707) 571-7560
FAX (707) 571-8929
Email: terrisu@sonic.net
AC,AN,CT,FP,NT,PM

SEBASTOPOL

Isaac Eliaz, MD
721 Jonive Rd.
Sebastopol, CA 95472
(707) 521-3376
FAX (707) 874-1815
Email: ieliaz@prodogy.net
GP

Norman Zucker, MD
867 Gravenstein Hwy. South
Sebastopol, CA 95472
(707) 823-6116
A,CT,DD,NT,MM,YS

SHERMAN OAKS

Rosamaria Ami Belli, MD
13481 Cheltenham Dr.
Sherman Oaks, CA 91423
NO REFERRALS

SONOMA

Jane-Ellen Heath, MD
853 Broadway
Sonoma, CA
(707) 938-0206
FAX (707) 938-0231
GP

STANTON

William J. Goldwag, MD
7499 Cerritos Ave.
Stanton, CA 90680
(714) 827-5180
CT,NT,PM

Donald Sharkoff, MD, PhD
8045 Cerritos Avenue
Stanton, CA 90680-0128
(714) 828-2444
FAX (714) 816-0529
GP

STUDIO CITY

Charles Law Jr., MD
3959 Laurel Canyon Blvd. Suite I
Studio City, CA 91604
(818) 761-1661
AC,BA,CT,GP,NT,PM

TEMPLETON

Carmelo A. Plateroti, DO,
BPCT
1111 Las Tablas Rd., #M
Templeton, CA 93465
(805) 434-2821
FAX (805) 434-2526
CT,DD,END,NT,PM,S,
Dermatology

TUSTIN

Leigh Erin Connealy, MD
14642 Newport Ave., #200
Tustin, CA 92780
(714) 669-4446
FAX (714) 669-4448
AC,BA,FP,END,MM, NT,PM

Allan Harvey Lane, MD, BPCT
17400 Irvine Blvd., #1
Tustin, CA 92780
(714) 544-9544
FAX (714) 544-9611
A,BA,CT,GYN,IM,NT,PM

Richard Lawrence Sellman,
MD
13422 Newport Avenue, Suite L
Sellman Health & Longevity
Tustin, CA 92780
(714) 544-1521
FAX (714) 544-3467
CT,END,FP,NT,PM,YS

UKIAH

Lawrence G. Foster, MD
230 B Hospital Drive
Ukiah, CA 95482
(707) 463-3502
CT,S

UPLAND

Bryan P. Chan, MD, BPCT
1148 San Bernardino Rd.
#E-102
Upland, CA 91786
(909) 920-3578
FAX (909) 949-1238
FP

VAN NUYS

Salvacion Lee, MD
15243 Vanowen St., #406
Van Nuys, CA 91405
(818) 785-7425
FAX (818) 785-7455
BA,CT,GP,HGL,NT,PM

VENTURA

Bob Young, MD
652 E. Main Street
Ventura, CA 93103
(805) 641-2022
CT,CD,DIA,DD,NY,PM,RHU

VISTA

Les Breitman, MD, BPCT
2023 W. Vista Way, Suite F
Vista, CA 92083
(760) 744-7766
FAX (760) 414-9933
anti_aging22@hotmail.com
CT,CD,DD,END,GER, NT,PM

WALNUT CREEK

Ingrid A. Bellwood, MD –
RETIRED
1300 Boulevard Way
Walnut Creek, CA 94595
NO REFERRALS

WOODLAND HILLS

A. Leonard Klepp, MD, APCT
22554 Ventura Blvd., #108
Woodland Hills, CA 91364
(818) 981-5511
FAX (818) 907-1468
CT,FP,PM,HGL,NT

COLORADO

ASPEN

Rob Krakovitz, MD
430 W. Main St.
Aspen, CO 81611
(970) 927-4394
A,CT,HGL,NT,PM,YS

AURORA

Terry A. Grossman, MD, APCT
3150 S. Peoria St., Unit H
Aurora, CO 80014
(303) 338-1323
FAX (303) 338-1324
CT,FP,NT,MM

BOULDER

Henry M. Johnston III, MD
7490 Clubhouse Rd., #103
Boulder, CO 80401
(303) 530-5555
FAX (303) 530-5522
CT,MM,DIA,NT,PM,YS

Ron Rosedale, MD, APCT
7490 Clubhouse Road
Boulder, CO 80301
(303) 530-5555
FAX (303) 530-5522
CT,CD,DIA,MN,NT

Michael A. Zeligs, MD, BPCT
1000 Alpine, #211
Boulder, CO 80304
(303) 442-5492
FAX (303) 447-3610
AN

COLORADO SPRINGS

George Juetersonke, DO, APCT
3525 American Drive
Colorado Springs, CO 80917
(719) 597-6075
FAX (719) 573-6529
A,AC,CT,HGL,NT,OSM,P

Joel Klein, MD
5455 N. Union Blvd., #201
Colorado Springs, CO 80918
(719) 457-0330
FAX (719) 457-0860
Email: jklein825@pol.net
FP

DENVER

Terry A. Grossman, MD, APCT
2025 South Xenia
Denver, CO 80231
(303) 233-4196
FAX (303) 233-4249
CT,FP,NT,MM

DURANGO

Ronald E. Wheeler, MD
2901 Main Avenue
Durango, CO 81301
(970) 259-4081
FAX (970) 247-3074
S,Oncology

GRAND JUNCTION

Joseph M. Wezensky, MD
2650 North Ave., Suite 101
Grand Junction, CO 81501
(970) 263-4660
FAX (970) 248-9519
CT,CD,PM,AA,Weight Reduction

GREENWOOD VILLAGE

Susanna S. Choi, MD
8200 E. Belleview Ave., #240E
Greenwood Village, CO 80111
(303) 721-1670
FAX (303) 721-8117
GYN,OBS

LAKEWOOD

Terry A. Grossman, MD, APCT
2801 Youngfield St., #117
Lakewood, CO 80401
(303) 233-4247
FAX (303) 233-4249
CT,FP,NT,MM

WESTMINSTER

Terry S. Friedmann, MD (H), APCT
P.O. Box 350128
Westminster, CO 80035-0128
NO REFERRALS

CONNECTICUT

BRIDGEPORT

Tadeusz A. Skowron, MD
50 Ridgefield Ave., #317
Bridgeport, CT 06610
(203) 368-1450
GP,IM

HAMDEN

Robert Lang, MD, PC
60 Washington Ave., #105
Hamden, CT 06518-3272
(203) 248-4362
FAX (203) 248-6933
DIA,END,HGL,MM,NT

MADISON

Robert Lang, MD, PC
11 Woodland Road
Madison, CT 06443
(203) 318-5264
DIA,END,HGL,MM,NT

MILFORD

Alan R. Cohen, MD, BPCT
67 Cherry Street
Milford, CT 06460
(203) 877-1936
CT,FP,NT,PD,PM,YS

RIDGEFIELD

Marcie Wolinsky-Friedland, MD
31 Bayley Avenue
Ridgefield, CT 06877
(203) 431-6165
FAX (203) 431-6167
CT,END,IM,PMR,P/S,RHU

STAMFORD

Henry C. Sobo, MD
122 Hoyt St., #D
Stamford, CT 06905
(203) 348-8805
FAX (203) 348-6398
A,BA,CD,CT,IM,NT,PM,HGL

TORRINGTON

Jerrold N. Finnie, MD, APCT
333 Kennedy Dr., #204
Torrington, CT 06790
(860) 489-8977
A,CT,CS,NT,RHI,YS

WATERBURY

Hamsa Jayaraj
47 Country Club Woods Circle
Waterbury, CT 06708
NO REFERRALS

DELAWARE

NEW CASTLE

Jeffrey K. Kerner, DO, BPCT
200 Bassett Ave.
New Castle, DE 19720
(302) 328-0669
FAX (302) 328-8937
Email: jkernerdo@aol.com
CT,FP,NT,OS,PM

DIST. OF COLUMBIA

WASHINGTON

Paul V. Beals, MD, BPCT
2639 Connecticut Avenue N.W.
Washington, DC 20008
(202) 332-0370
CT,FP,NT,PM

George H. Mitchell, MD
2639 Connecticut Ave. N.W.,
Suite C-100
Washington, DC 20008
(202) 265-41111
A,NT

Aldo M. Rosemblat, MD, APCT
5225 Wisconsin Ave. N.W., #401
Washington, DC 20015
(202) 237-7000
FAX (202) 237-0017
AC,S

FLORIDA
APOPKA

Allan Zubkin, MD
424 N. Park Ave.
Apopka, FL 32712
(407) 886-0611
FAX (407) 886-2817
Email: azmd@aol.com
GP,CS,CT

AVENTURA

Sylvan R. Lewis, MD
20335 Biscayne Blvd., #L-11
Aventura, FL 33180
(305) 705-0106
FAX (305) 705-0109
CD,IM,NT

BEVERLY HILLS

James Lemire, MD, BPCT
4065 N. Lecanto Hwy., #100
Beverly Hills, FL 34465
(352) 527-6840
FAX (352) 527-6843
Email: jlemire@hitter.net
FP,AA

BOCA RATON

Leonard Haimes, MD
7300 N. Federal Hwy., #100
Boca Raton, FL 33487-1631
(561) 995-8484
FAX (561) 995-7773
A,BA,CT,IM,NT,PM

Robert D. Willix Jr., MD
1515 S. Federal Hwy., #306
Boca Raton, FL 33432
(561) 362-0724
FAX (561) 362-9924
CD,HGL,MM,NT,PM,PMR

BONITA SPRINGS

Stepehn Kaskie, MD
#2100–3501 Health Center Blvd.
Bonita Springs, FL 39135
(941) 948-2000
FAX (941) 948-2058
Email: stevedoc1@aol.com
FP

Dean R. Silver, MD
9240 Bonita Beach Rd., #2215
Gulfcoast Longevity and
Wellness Center
Bonita Springs, FL 34135
(941) 949-0101
FAX (941) 949-4334
CD,DD,END,IM,PM,YS

BOYNTON BEACH

Kenneth Lee, MD
1325 S. Congress, #208
Boynton Beach, FL 33426
(561) 736-8806
CD,GER,IM,NT,GP

BRADENTON

Eteri Melnikov, MD, APCT
116 Manatee Ave. East
Bradenton, FL 34208
(941) 748-7943

CD,CT,DIA,GP,PM,YS

CASSELBERRY

Jeffrey Mueller, MD, BPCT
1455 S. Semoran Blvd., #299
Casselberry, FL 32707
(407) 657-2433
FAX (407) 657-5823
AC,AN,GP,PM

CLEARWATER

Donald J. Carrow, MD
4908 Creekside Dr., #A
Clearwater, FL 34620
(727) 573-3775
FAX (727) 556-0082
Email: htyh@mindspring.com
AN,CD,CT,DD,MM,NT,PM

John P. Lenhart, MD, BPCT
2250 State Road 580
Clearwater, FL 33761
(727) 526-0600
FAX (727) 799-8024
AC,BA,NT,PM,PMR,P/S

David Minkoff, MD
301 Turner Street
Clearwater, FL 33756
(727) 442-5612
CT,NT,PM,CD,PMR

David M. Wall, MD
1749 Long Bow Lane
Clearwater, FL 33764
(727) 724-0135
FAX (727) 724-0129
AN,AC,CT,DD,NT,PM

CORAL SPRINGS

Jerald H. Ratner, MD
9750 N.W. 33rd St., #211
Coral Springs, FL 33065
(954) 752-9450
FAX (954) 752-9888
P

Anthony J. Sancetta, DO, BPCT
2041 University Drive
Coral Springs, FL 33071
(954) 344-4343
Email: tsancetta@pol.net
CT,GP,NT,OS,PM,PMR

CRAWFORDVILLE

Royce V. Jackson, MD, APCT
39 Lighthouse Point
Crawfordville, FL 32327
NO REFERRALS

FORT LAUDERDALE

David J. Blyweiss, MD
100 S.E. 15th Ave.
Fort Lauderdale, FL 33301
(954) 763-1230
FAX (954) 763-1238
GP

Cristino C. Enriquez, MD, BPCT
767 S. State Road 7
Fort Lauderdale, FL 33317
(954) 583-3335
FAX (954) 463-8006
CD,CT,IM,PM,PUD,R

Bach A. McComb, DO, ND, PhD
2545 E. Sunrise Blvd., #202
Fort Lauderdale, FL 33304
(954) 661-2225
OS,CT,P/S,NT,PM,PMR

FORT MYERS

Robert A. Didonato, MD
3443 Hancock Bridge Pkwy., #301
N. Ft. Myers, FL 33903
(941) 997-8800
FAX (941) 997-7706
Email: BobD@OLSUSA.com
CT,NT,GP,P/S

Gayle Kesselman, MD
1342 Colonial Blvd., #K-116
Fort Myers, FL 33907
(941) 939-9898
FAX (941) 275-7030
P

John R. Pletincks II, MD, BPCT
6314 Whiskey Creek Drive
Fort Myers, FL 33919
(941) 590-6332
FAX (941) 433-2331
CT,DD,END,S,Anti-Aging,P/S

Gary L. Pynkel, DO, APCT
3840 Colonial Blvd., #1
Fort Myers, FL 33912
(941) 278-3377
FAX (941) 278-3702
CT,FP,GP,OSM,PM

GAINESVILLE

Robert Erickson, MD
905 N.W. 56th Terrace, Suite B
Gainesville, FL 32605
(352) 331-5138
FAX (352) 331-9399
Email: raericksonmd@ez-tel.com
FP,PM

Hanoch Talmor, MD
4421 N.W. 39th Ave., Bldg. 2-1
Gainesville, FL 32606-7214
(352) 377-0015
FAX (352) 378-1895
Email: talmor@msn.com
CT,HOM,NT,YS

HOLIDAY

Robert J. Hannum, DO, BPCT
2216 US Hwy. 19
Holiday, FL 34691
(727) 937-6428
CT,FP,GER,OS

HOLLYWOOD

Herbert Pardell, DO, APCT
4330 Sheridan Street, #102
Hollywood, FL 33021
(954) 987-4455
FAX (954) 964-7342
Email: PARDELL1@aol.com
CT,DD,IM,MM,NT,PM

HOMOSASSA SPRINGS

Carlos F. Gonzalez, MD, APCT
7989 So. Suncoast Blvd.
Homosassa Springs, FL 32646
(352) 382-2900
FAX (352) 382-1633
A,CD,CS,END,PMR,RHU

INDIALANTIC

Glen Wagner, MD, BPCT
121 – 6th Ave.
Indialantic, FL 32903
(407) 723-5915
A,AC,CT,GP,NT,YS

INDIAN HARBOUR BEACH

Daniel B. Hammond, MD
1413 South Patrick Drive
Indian Harbour Beach, FL 32937
(407) 777-9923
FAX (407) 777-4707
DIA,FP,GP,HGL,NT,PM

JACKSONVILLE

Norman S. Cohen, MD, APCT
5150 Belfort Road, Bldg. 400
The Vein Clinic & Longevity Center
Jacksonville, FL 32256-6026
(904) 296-0900
FAX (904) 296-8346
OBS,GYN,Altern. Med.

Sanford Z. Pollak, DO
4131 S. University Blvd., #11
Jacksonville, FL 32216
(904) 636-7755
FAX (904) 636-5885
OS,P/S,Pain Mngt.

KEY BISCAYNE

Sam Baxas, MD
50 West Mashta Dr., #3
Key Biscayne, FL 33149
(305) 361-9249
FAX (305) 361-2179
AC,AU,CT,GP,BA,FP

KISSIMMEE

Carmelita Bamba-Dagani, MD
1318 West Oak St.
Kissimmee, FL 34741
(407) 931-1887
FAX (407) 931-2056
AN,AC,AU,CT,Pain Mngt.

LADY LAKE

Nelson Kraucak, MD, APCT
8985 N.E. 134th Avenue
Lady Lake, FL 32159
(352) 750-4333
FAX (352) 750-2023
AC,AR,CT,NT,FP,Prolotherapy

LAKE CITY

Barnie Vanzant, MD, BPCT
503 S. Hernando St.
Lake City, FL 32025
(904) 752-9222
FP

LAKE MARY

Diab Ashrap, MD
3859 Lake Emma Rd.
Lake Mary, FL 32746
(407) 805-9222
FAX (407) 444-5299
ashrapdiab@hotmail.com
IM

LAKE WORTH

Sherri W. Pinsley, DO
2290 – 10th Ave. North, #605
Lake Worth, FL 33461
(561) 547-2770
CT,DD,GP,NT,OS,PMR

LAKELAND

Harold Robinson, MD
4406 S. Florida Ave., Suite 27
Lakeland, FL 33803
(941) 646-5088
CT,FP,GP,HGL,NT,PM

S. Todd Robinson, MD, APCT
4406 S. Florida Ave., Suite 30
Lakeland, FL 33803
(941) 646-5088
CT,FP,GP,HGL,NT,PM

LAUDERHILL

Herbert R. Slavin, MD, APCT
7200 W. Commercial Blvd.,
Suite #210
Lauderhill, FL 33319
(954) 748-4991
FAX (954) 748-5022
Email: drslavin@aol.com
CT,DIA,DD,GER,IM,NT

LECANTO

Azael P. Borromeo, MD, APCT
2653 N. Lecanto Hwy.
Lecanto, FL 34461
(352) 527-9555
FAX (352) 527-2609
BA,GP,PATHOLOGY,S

LONGWOOD

Donald E. Colbert, MD
1908 Booth Circle
Longwood, FL 32750
(407) 331-7007
FAX (407) 331-5777
FP

Robert J. Rogers, MD
2170 West State Road 434, #190
Longwood, FL 32779
(407) 682-5222
FAX (407) 682-5274
A,CT,NT,PM,HGL,YS

MAITLAND

Joya Lynn Schoen, MD, BPCT
341 N. Maitland Ave., Suite 200
Maitland, FL 32751
(407) 644-2729
FAX (407) 644-1205
CD,CT,GP,HOM,MM,NT,OME,YS

MARCO ISLAND

Richard Saitta, MD
1010 N. Barfield Dr.
Marco Island, FL 34145
(941) 642-8488
AC,CT,HO,IM,NT,PM

MELBOURNE

Neil Ahner, MD, APCT
1270 N. Wickham Road
Melbourne, FL 32935
(407) 253-2009
FAX (407) 253-5561
Email: DocAhner@aol.com
CT,NT,PM

Rajiv Chandra, MD, BPCT
20 E. Melbourne Ave. #104
Melbourne, FL 32901
(407) 951-7404
CD,CS,GP,IM,NT,PM

MIAMI

Stefano DiMauro, MD
16695 N.E. 10th Avenue
N. Miami Beach, FL 33162
(305) 940-6474
FAX (305) 944-8601
A,CT,DIA,FP,NT,PMR

Cristino C. Enriquez, MD, BPCT
8229 South Dixie Highway
Miami, FL 33143
(305) 668-0038
FAX (305) 668-9546
CD,CT,IM,PM,PUD,R

Joseph G. Godorov, DO
9055 S.W. 87th Ave., Suite 307
Miami, FL 33176
(305) 595-0671
CT,END,FP,HGL,NT,PM

Alvaro H. Skupin, MD
8360 S.W. 8th St.
Miami, FL 33144
(305) 265-8929
IM,PUD, Sleep Disorders

Wynne A. Steinsnyder, DO
17291 N.E. 19th Avenue
N. Miami Beach, FL 33162
(305) 947-0618
FAX (305) 940-1345
OS,GP,PMR,S,Urology

Ivonne F. Torre-Coya, MD
10534 S.W. 8th
Miami, FL 33174
(305) 223-0132
FAX (305) 553-6488
BA,CT,FP,HGL,YS

MILTON

William Watson, MD
5536 Stewart Street
Milton, FL 32570
(850) 623-3836
FAX (850) 623-2201
BA,GP,S,CT,PM,WR

MOUNT DORA

Jack E. Young, MD, PhD, APCT
2260 W. Old Hwy. 441
Mount Dora, FL 32757
(352) 385-4400
FAX (352) 385-4402
Email: jyoungmd@mpinet.net
CT,GP,MM,NT,OME,PM

NAPLES

David Perlmutter, MD
800 Goodlette Rd. N., #270
Naples, FL 33940
(941) 649-7400
FAX (941) 649-6370
DD,END,FP,NT,PM,Neurology

John R. Pletincks II, MD, BPCT
501 Goodlette Road North, #302
Naples, FL 33940
(941) 434-8553
FAX (941) 433-2331
CT,DD,END,S,Anti-Aging,P/S

NEW SMYRNA BEACH

William Campbell Douglass, III, MD, APCT
2111 Ocean Drive
New Smyrna Beach, FL 32169
NO REFERRALS
Email: turtletracks@cfl.rr.com

OCALA

George Graves, DO
11512 County Road 316
P.O. Box 2220
Ocala (Ft. McCoy), FL 32134
(352) 236-2525
FAX (352) 236-8610
A,AR,BA,CT,GP,OS

John P. Salerno, DO
3240 SW 34th Street, Apt. 921
Ocala, FL 34474
(352) 237-1103
FAX (352) 861-5447
Email: doctorsalerno@aol.com
FP,OS,PM

ORANGE CITY

Travis L. Herring, MD
106 West Fern Dr.
Orange City, FL 32763
(904) 775-0525
CT,FP,HOM,IM

ORMOND BEACH

Hana Chaim, DO
595 W. Granada Blvd., #D
Ormond Beach, FL 32174
(904) 672-9000
A,CT,Env. Med.,FP, Sclerotherapy

PACE

P.K. Garg, MD
5553 Hwy. 90
Pace, FL 32571
(850) 995-8811
FAX (850) 995-8810
FP

PALM BEACH GARDENS

Neil Ahner, MD, APCT
10333 N. Military Trail, Suite A
Palm Beach Gardens, FL 33410
(561) 630-3696
FAX (561) 630-1991
Email: DocAhner@aol.com
CT,NT,PM

PALM HARBOR

Glenn Chapman, MD
34621 U.S. Highway 19, North
Palm Harbor Physicians
Walk-In-Clinic
Palm Harbor, FL 34684
(727) 786-1661
FAX (727) 785-3783
CT,FP,GP,NT,PM

Carlos M. Garcia, MD, APCT
36555 U.S. Hwy. 19 North
Palm Harbor, FL 34684
(727) 771-9669
FAX (727) 771-8071
AN,CD,CT,IM,PM,Pain Mgmt.

PANAMA CITY

Naima Abdel-Ghany,
MD,PhD, APCT
340 W. 23rd Street, Suite K
Panama City, FL 32405
(850) 872-8122
FAX (850) 872-9925
A,CD,CT,IM,PUD,PH,PM,
Anti-Aging Med.

James W. De Ruiter, MD
2202 State Ave., #311
Panama City, FL 32405
(850) 747-4963
FAX (850) 747-0074
OBS-GYN

Samir M.A. Yassin, MD
516 S. Tyndall Pkwy., #202
Panama City, FL 32404
(850) 763-0464
doctor.medscape.com/yassin
BA,CT,DD,DIA,GP,PM

PENSACOLA

Ward Dean, MD
P.O. Box 11097
Pensacola, FL 32524
NO REFERRALS

PLANTATION

Adam Frent, DO
1741 N. University Drive
Plantation, FL 33322
(954) 474-1617
FAX (954) 472-1631
CT,DIA,DD,FP,GER,PM

Alvin Stein, MD
4101 N.W. 4 St., #S-401
Plantation, FL 33317
(954) 581-8585
FAX (954) 581-5580
CT,PMR,P/S

PORT ST. LUCIE

Steven Everett, MD
1837 Port St. Lucoe Blvd.
Port St. Lucie, FL 34957
(561) 398-8884
FAX (561) 398-9898
Email: severettmd@aol.com
PM,HO

PUNTA GORDA

James Coy, MD, BPCT
310 Nesbit St.,
P.O. Box 511315
Punta Gorda, FL 33951
(941) 575-8080
FAX (941) 575-8108
A,CT,GP

SARASOTA

W. Frederic Harvey, MD
3982 Bee Ridge Rd., Bldg. H, #J
Sarasota, FL 34239
(941) 929-9355
GER,IM,MM,NT,PM

Ronald E. Wheeler, MD
The Sarasota City Center
1819 Main Street, #401
Sarasota, FL 34236
(941) 957-0007
S,Oncology

SPRING HILL

Nabil Habib, MD, BPCT
11097 Hearth Road
Spring Hill, FL 34608
(352) 683-1166
FAX (352) 683-2902
S

Calin V. Pop, MD
4215 Rachel Boulevard
Spring Hill, FL 34607
(352) 597-2240
FAX (352) 597-2990
BA,CT,GP,IM

ST. PETERSBURG

John P. Lenhart, MD, BPCT
5763 – 38th Ave. N.
St. Petersburg, FL 33710
(727) 526-0600
FAX (727) 345-0928
AC,BA,NT,PM,PMR,P/S

Ray Wunderlich Jr., MD, APCT
1152 – 94th Ave. North
St. Petersburg, FL 33702
(727) 822-3612
FAX (727) 578-1370
Email: wctr@gte.net
A,CT,DD,NT,YS,HGL,MM

STUART

Neil Ahner, MD, APCT
705 North Federal Hwy.
Stuart, FL 34994
(561) 692-9200
FAX (561) 692-9888
Email: DocAhner@aol.com
CT,NT,PM

Sherri W. Pinsley, DO
7000 S.E. Federal Hwy.
Suite #302
Stuart, FL 34997
(561) 220-1697
FAX (561) 220-7332
CT,DD,GP,NT,OS,PMR

SUNNY ISLES BEACH

Martin Dayton, DO, APCT
18600 Collins Ave.
Sunny Isles Beach, FL 33160
(305) 931-8484
FAX (305) 936-1849
Email: mddomddo@pol.net
CT,FP,GER,NT,OSM,PM

TALLAHASSEE

William Watson, MD
1630-A North Plaza Drive
Tallahassee, FL 32308
(850) 878-2888
BA,CT,GP,S,CT,PM,WR

TAMARAC

George A. Lustig, MD
7401 N. University Dr., #101
Tamarac, FL 33321
(954) 724-0099
FAX (954) 724-0070
CD,IM,NT

TAMPA

Jean Allen, DO
4543 S. Manhattan Ave., #103
Tampa, FL 33611
(813) 831-8888
A,FP,GYN,NT,PM,NHR

Carlos M. Garcia, MD, APCT
4710 Havana Ave., #107
Tampa, FL 33616
(813) 350-0140
FAX (813) 350-0713
AN,CD,CT,IM,PM,Pain Mgmt.

Eugene H. Lee, MD
1804 W. Kennedy Blvd. #A
Tampa, FL 33606
(813) 251-3089
FAX (813) 251-5668
AC,CT,NT,PM,GP,HGL,
Prolotherapy

TAVARES

Nelson Kraucak, MD, BPCT
204 N. Texas Avenue
Tavares, FL 32778
(352) 742-1116
FAX (352) 742-8288
AC,AR,CT,NT,Neural Therapy

VENICE

Arlene Martone, MD
4140 Woodmere Park Blvd., #2
Venice, FL 34293
(941) 408-9838

VERO BEACH

Neil Ahner, MD, APCT
717 17th Street
Vero Beach, FL 32960
(561) 978-0057
FAX (561) 978-9652
Email: DocAhner@aol.com
CT,NT,PM

John Song, MD, BPCT
1360 U.S. 1, #1
Vero Beach, FL 32960
(561) 770-2070
FAX (561) 569-1593
CT,FP,GP,IM,NT,PM,S

WEST PALM BEACH

Daniel N. Tucker, MD
1411 N. Flagler Dr., #6700
West Palm Beach, FL 33401
(561) 835-0055
FAX (561) 835-1742
A,CS,PUD,RHI

GEORGIA

ATLANTA

Earl L. Alderman, MD
1938 Peachtree Rd., #101
Atlanta, GA 30309
(404) 351-1151
CT,GP,S

Rhett Bergeron, MD
4370 Georgetown Square
Atlanta, GA 30338
(770) 390-0012
FAX (770) 457-9440
americanwellnessinstitute@msn
.com
CT,MM,NT,PM,P/S,YS

M. Truett Bridges, Jr., MD,
BPCT
4920 Roswell Rd., #35
Atlanta, GA 30342
(404) 843-8880
FAX (404) 843-8687
AN,AC,AU,CT,PM,NT

Stephen B. Edelson, MD
3833 Roswell Rd., #110
Atlanta, GA 30342
(404) 841-0088
FAX (404) 841-6416
Email: sbedelson@pol.com
CT,NT,FP, Env. Med.,PM

Milton Fried, MD, APCT
4426 Tilly Mill Road
Atlanta, GA 30360
(770) 451-4857
FAX (770) 451-8492
A,CT,IM,NT,PM,PO

Susan E. Kolb, MD
4370 Georgetown Square
Atlanta, GA 30338
(770) 457-4677
FAX (770) 457-4428
millennium_hc@yahoo.com
S,HO,CT

AUGUSTA

William J. Lee, MD, BPCT
#2N (Le Pavilion Mall)
106 Pleasant Home Rd.
Augusta, GA 30907
(706) 869-0069
CT,S

BREMER

Rhett Bergeron, MD
200 Tallapoosa Street
Bremer, GA 30110
(770) 537-4445
FAX (770) 537-1747
americanwellnessinstitute@msn
.com
CT,MM,NT,PM,P/S,YS

BRUNSWICK

Ralph G. Ellis Jr., MD, APCT
158 Scranton Connector
Brunswick, GA 31525
(912) 280-0304
FAX (912) 280-0601
Email: rgellis@darientel.net
CT,DD,NT,PM,CD, Oxidative
Therapy

CANTON

William Early, MD
320 Hospital Rd.
Canton, GA 30114
(770) 479-5535
FAX (770) 720-3294
IM,GE

CARTERSVILLE

Claude R. Poliak, MD, BPCT
13 Bowens Court
Cartersville, GA 30120
(770) 607-0220
FAX (770) 607-0208
OPH,CT,NT,A,Env. Med.,
Anti-Aging

CLAYTON

William J. Lee, MD, BPCT
P.O. Box 229
145 Rickman Street
Clayton, GA 30525
(706) 782-4044
FAX (706) 782-4030
CT,S

COLUMBUS

William J. Lee, MD, BPCT
9249 Veterans Parkway
Columbus, GA 31820
(706) 653-2247
CT,S

Jan McBarron, MD
2904 Macon Rd.
Columbus, GA 31906
(706) 322-4073
FAX (706) 323-4786
BA,NT,PM

FORT OGLETHORPE

Charles C. Adams, MD, BPCT
3047 Battlefield Pkwy.
Fort Oglethorpe, GA 30742
(706) 861-7377
FAX (706) 861-7922
IM,CT,NT,A,Anti-Aging Med.

GAINESVILLE

John L. Givogre, MD, BPCT
530 Springs Street
Gainesville, GA 30501
(770) 503-7222
AN,CT,PMR

Kathryn Herndon, MD
530 Spring St.
Gainesville, GA 30503
(770) 503-7222
AC,AU,CT,NT,OS,PMR

LAGRANGE

Earl L. Alderman, MD
302 South Greenwood St.
LaGrange, GA 30240
(706) 884-8360
FAX (706) 884-0258
CT,GP,S

LAWRENCEVILLE

Kathy Roberti-Kiepura, MD
911 Duluth Hwy. N.W., #B-6
Lawrenceville, GA 30043
(770) 339-1311
FAX (770) 339-3608
NT,PD,PM

MACON

James T. Alley, MD
2518 Riverside Dr.
Macon, GA 31204
(478) 745-3727
or (800) 547-9743
CT,NT,Horm. Repl., Rehab

MARIETTA

Ralph Lee, MD
110 Lewis Dr., Suite B
Marietta, GA 30060
(770) 423-0064
FAX (770) 423-9827
CT,GP,NT,PM,YS

NORCROSS

Mark Stallman, MD
200 Merchant Drive, #204
Norcross, GA 30093
(770) 908-0468
FAX (770) 908-0469
Email: mark@aol.com
IM,FP,BA,PM

OGLETHORPE

Elwin Glynn Taunton, DO,
BPCT
100 Riverview Lane
P.O. Box 1069
Oglethorpe, GA 31068
(912) 472-2550
FAX (912) 472-2555
CT,FP,GER,OS,PM, Sclerotherapy

ROSWELL

Marcia V. Byrd, MD
11050 Crabapple Rd., #105-B
Roswell, GA 30075
(770) 587-1711
A,CT,GP,NT,PM,YS

SMYRNA

Donald Ruesink, MD
1004 Lincoln Trace Cir. S.E.
Smyrna, GA 30080
(770) 818-9908
CT,NT

William Stafano, MD –
RETIRED
645 Windy Hill Rd.
Smyrna, GA 30080
NO REFERRALS

STOCKBRIDGE

Rhett Bergeron, MD
115 Eagle Spring Dr., #A
Stockbridge, GA 30281
(770) 474-4422
FAX (770) 474-7702
americanwellnessinstitute@msn
.com
CT,MM,NT,PM,P/S,YS

Michael Rowland, MD
130 Eagle Springs Court, Suite A
Stockbridge, GA 30281
(770) 507-2930
FAX (770) 507-0837
CT,FP,DIA,NT,WR,CD

T.R. Shantha, MD, PhD
115 Eagle Spring Dr.
Stockbridge, GA 32081
(770) 474-4029
FAX (770) 474-2038
Email: shantha35@aol.com
nesthisiology

WETUMPKA

Mark Hayden, MD
776297 Tallahassee Hwy.
Wetumpka, GA 36092
(334) 514-1910
FAX (334) 567-3025
GP

HAWAII

HONOLULU

Chol Bae Kim, MD
1441 Kapiolani Blvd., #2020
Honolulu, HI 96814
(808) 941-3997
FAX (808) 941-3933
FP,PM

Frederick Lam, MD, APCT
1270 Queen Emma St., #501
Honolulu, HI 96813
(808) 537-3311
FAX (808) 946-0378
Email: hamkhgg@aloha.net
A,AC,CT,FP,HGL

Keith Tonoki, MD
1301 Punchbowl Street
Honolulu, HI 96813
(808) 547-4271
FAX (808) 547-4045
Email: ktonoki@queens.com
IM, Pathology

KAILUA-KONA

JoAnne Lombardi, MD
76-997 S. Pakalakala Place
Kailua-Kona, HI 96740
(808) 327-2952

KAPAA, KAUAI

Thomas R. Yarema, MD, BPCT
4504 Kukui St., #13
Kapaa, Kauai, HI 96741
(808) 823-0994
FAX (808) 823-0995
Email: namastay@gte.net
FP,CT,GP,NT,PM,S

PAHOA

Alan D. Thal, MD
P.O. Box 403
Pahoa, HI 96778
(808) 982-7899
FAX (808) 982-6770
A,AC,HYP,NT,PD

IDAHO

NAMPA

Stephen Thornburgh, DO, APCT
824 – 17th Ave. So.
Nampa, ID 83651
(208) 466-3517
AC,CT,HOM,OS

ILLINOIS

ARLINGTON HEIGHTS

Terrill K. Haws, DO
121 So. Wilke Road, Suite 111
Arlington Heights, IL 60005
(847) 577-9451
FAX (847) 577-8601
CT,DD,FP,GP,OSM

AURORA

Thomas Hesselink, MD
888 So. Edgelawn Dr., Suite 1743
Aurora, IL 60506
(630) 844-0011
FAX (630) 844-0500
A,CT,GP,NT,PM, Candida

BELVIDERE

Thomas Hesselink, MD
6413 Logan Ave., #104
Belvidere, IL 61008
(815) 547-8187
FAX (815) 547-6461
A,CT,GP,NT,PM, Candida

Oscar I. Ordonez, MD
6413 Logan Ave., #104
Belvidere, IL 61008
(815) 547-8187
FAX (815) 544-3114
A,CT,IM,NT,PM

BRAIDWOOD

Bernard Milton, MD
233 E. Reed St.
Braidwood, IL 60408
(815) 458-6700
AC,AU,CT,FP,HGL,YS

CHICAGO

Alan F. Bain, DO
30 N. Michigan Ave., #1410
Chicago, IL 60602
(312) 236-7010
AC,CT,IM,NT,OS

David Edelberg, MD
2522 N. Lincoln Avenue
Chicago, IL 60614
(773) 296-6700
FAX (773) 296-1131
AC,DD,CT,IM,NT,YS

Razvan Rentea, MD
3525 W. Peterson, Suite 611
Chicago, IL 60659
(773) 583-7793
FAX (773) 583-7796
GP,MM,PM

ELK GROVE VILLAGE

Zofia Szymanska, MD
850 Biesterfield Rd., #4006
Elk Grove Village, IL 60007
(847) 437-4418
GYN,OBS,YS,PM,END,NT

GENEVA

Richard E. Hrdlicka, MD
302 Randall Rd., #206
Geneva, IL 60134
(630) 232-1900
A,BA,FP,NT,PM,YS

HAZEL CREST

Prakash G. Sane, MD
17680 South Kedzie Ave.
Hazel Crest, IL 60429
(708) 799-2499
FAX (708) 799-4093
FP

HOFFMAN ESTATES

Susan Busse, MD
Governor's Place Medical Bldg.
2260 W. Higgins Rd., #202
Hoffman Estates, IL 60195
(847) 781-7500
FAX (847) 781-7502
A,CT,DD,END,NT,PM,FP

METAMORA

Robert E. Thompson, MD
205 S. Englewood Drive
Metamora, IL 61548
(309) 367-2321
FAX (309) 367-2324
OB/GYN,FP,CT

OAK PARK

Paul J. Dunn, MD
715 Lake Street
Oak Park, IL 60301
(708) 383-3800
FAX (708) 383-3445
Email: pjkddunn@aol.com
CT,HGL,NT,OSM,PM,YS

Ross A. Hauser, MD
715 Lake Street, Suite 600
Oak Park, IL 60301
(708) 848-7789
FAX (708) 848-7763
drhauser@caringmedical.com
AN,CT,DD,NT,PMR,RHU,
Prolotherapy

SCHAUMBURG

Joseph Mercola, DO
1443 W. Schaumburg Rd., #250
Schaumburg, IL 60194
(847) 985-1777
A,AR,CT,GP,NT,RHU,YS

WHEATON

Fred J. Schultz, MD
529 W. Roosevelt Rd.
Wheaton, IL 60187
(630) 933-9700
FAX (630) 933-9724
A,END,FP,NT,PM,YS

INDIANA

BLOOMINGTON

Michael W. Kane, MD
722 W. 2nd Street
Bloomington, IN 47403
(812) 331-1601
FAX (812) 331-1603
AC,MM,PM,P,PO

CLARKSVILLE

George Wolverton, MD, APCT
647 Eastern Blvd.
Clarksville, IN 47129
(812) 282-4309
CD,CT,FP,GYN,PM,PD

EVANSVILLE

Larry W. Banyash, MD, APCT
611 Harriett Street, #402
Evansville, IN 47710
(812) 421-6920
FAX (812) 421-6925
BA,CT,FP,NT,PM,PMR (Sports
Medicine)

Joseph Waling, MD
8601 N. Kentucky Ave., Suite G
Evansville, IN 47725
(812) 867-9800
FAX (812) 867-4720
PMR,CT,OSM,P/S,R

HUNTINGTON

Thomas J. Ringenberg, DO,
BPCT
941 Etwa Avenue
Huntington, IN 46750
(219) 356-9400
FAX (219) 356-4254
FP,OS,NT,PM

INDIANAPOLIS

Robert S. Daly, MD
1250 E. County Line Rd., #2
Indianapolis, IN 46227
(317) 885-3677
FAX (317) 885-3678
FP,IM,PUD,Critical Care

David A. Darbro, MD
8202 Clearvista Parkway,
Bldg. 7, #A
Indianapolis, IN 46256
(317) 913-3000
FAX (317) 913-1000
drdarbro@abchealth.com
A,AR,CT,DD,FP,PM

David R. Decatur, MD
8925 N. Meridan, #150
Indianapolis, IN 46260
(317) 818-8925
AC,CD,CT,HYP,NT,PM

Samia T. Mercho, MD
11216 Fall Creek Rd.
Indianapolis, IN 46256
(317) 595-8823
FAX (317) 595-4697
MerchoTawilmed@aol.com
IM

JEFFERSONVILLE

H. Wayne Mayhue, MD
207 Sparks Ave. #301
Jeffersonville, IN 47130
(812) 288-7169
FAX (812) 288-2861
OB-GYN

LAFAYETTE

Charles Turner, MD, BPCT
2433 S. 9th Street
Lafayette, IN 47909
(765) 471-1100
FAX (765) 471-1009
FP,A,CT,P/S,NT,HO

LYNN

David Chopra, MD
P.O. Box 636
428 South Main St.
Lynn, IN 47355
(317) 874-2411
AC,BA,CT,DD,GER,IM

MERRILLVILLE

Joel F. Lopez, MD
5495 Broadway
Merrillville, IN 46410
(219) 985-5500
FAX (219) 985-5510
CT,GP

MIDDLEBURY

Douglas W. Elliott, MD, BPCT
801 – 8 W. Wayne
Middlebury, IN 46540
(219) 825-4312
FAX (219) 825-4155
FP,NT

MOORESVILLE

Richard N. Halstead, DO
215 E. High St.
Mooresville, IN 46158
(317) 831-0853
FAX (317) 831-0864
GP

NO. MANCHESTER

Marvin D. Dziabis, MD
107 West Seventh Street
No. Manchester, IN 46962
(219) 982-2352
FAX (219) 982-1700
Email: mdziabis@ctlnet.com
AR,CD,CT,NT,HOM,YS

PARKER CITY

Oscar I. Ordonez, MD
218 S. Main Street
Parker City, IN 47368
(765) 468-6337
A,CT,IM,NT,PM

SOUTH BEND

Keim T. Houser, MD
515 N. Lafayette Blvd.
South Bend, IN 46601
(219) 232-2037
GYN,OBS

Anne L. Kempf, DO
1202 Lincolnway East
South Bend, IN 46601
(219) 232-5892
AU,CT,GP,OS

VALPARAISO

Myrna D. Trowbridge, DO
850-C Marsh St.
Valparaiso, IN 46383
(219) 462-3377
AC,AR,CT,FP,NT,OSM

KANSAS

ANDOVER

William C. Simon, DO
324 W. Central, #E
Andover, KS 67002
(316) 733-4494
FAX (316) 733-5792
CT,CD,NT,YS,AC

COFFEYVILLE

J. E. Block, MD
1501 W. 4th
Coffeyville, KS 67337
(316) 251-2400
FAX (316) 251-1619
Email: drblock@hit.net
CD,IM

GARDEN CITY

Terry Hunsberger, DO
603 N. 5th Street
Garden City, KS 67846
(316) 275-3760
FAX (316) 275-3704
BA,CT,FP,NT,OSM,PM

HAYS

Roy N. Neil, MD
105 West 13th
Hays, KS 67601
(913) 628-8341
BA,CD,CT,DD,NT,PM

KANSAS CITY

Jeanne A. Drisko, MD,BPCT
3901 Rainbow Blvd.
Kansas City, KS 66160
(913) 588-6208
FAX (913) 588-6271
Email: jdrisko@kumc.edu
GP,NT,PM,R

LIBERAL

Bob Sager, MD
2130 N. Kansas Ave.
Liberal, KS 67901
(316) 626-5060
FAX (316) 626-7993
AC,CT,FP,NT,YS

KENTUCKY

BEREA

Edward K. Atkinson, MD
P.O. Box 57
Berea, KY 40403
(606) 925-2252
FAX (606) 925-2252
AN,CT

PROSPECT

Kirk Morgan, MD, FACAM,
APCT
9105 U.S. Hwy. 42
Prospect, KY 40059
(502) 228-0156
FAX (502) 228-0512
CD,CT,FP,MM,NT,YS

SOMERSET

Stephen S. Kiteck, MD
600 Bogle St.
Somerset, KY 42501
(606) 677-0459
FP,IM,PD,PM

LOUISIANA

ALEXANDRIA

James W. Welch, MD
4300 Parliament Dr.
Alexandria, LA 71303
(318) 448-0221
S

BATON ROUGE

Rhett Bergeron, MD
7964-F Wrenwood Blvd.
Baton Rouge, LA 70809
(225) 802-2578
CT,MM,NT,PM,P/S,YS

Stephanie F. Cave, MD, BPCT
7777 Hennessy, #101
Baton Rouge, LA 70808-4363
(225) 767-7433
FAX (225) 767-4641
FP,A,NT,PM,YS,DD

Scott J. Daigle, MD, BPCT
8754 Goodwood Blvd.
Baton Rouge, LA 70806
(225) 927-6400
FAX (225) 923-1742
FP

BELLE CHASSE

Lawrence A. Giambelluca,
MD
8200 Wighway 23
Belle Chasse, LA 70037
(504) 398-1100
FAX (504) 398-1030
CT,FP

CHALMETTE

Saroj T. Tampira, MD
800 W. Virtue St., Suite 207
Chalmette, LA 70043
(504) 277-8991
FAX (504) 277-8997
CD,DD,DIA,IM

COVINGTON

Roy M. Montalbano, MD –
RETIRED
224 Tchefuncle Drive
Covington, LA 70433-4808
NO REFERRALS

LAFAYETTE

Sydney Crackower, MD
701 Robley Dr., #100
Lafayette, LA 70503
(337) 988-4116
CT,FP,GER

Sangeeta Shah, MD
211 E. Kaliste Saloom
Lafayette, LA 70508
(337) 235-1166
FAX (337) 235-1168
BA,DIA,HGL,NT,PM

MANDEVILLE

James P. Carter, MD, APCT
4408 Hwy. 22
Mandeville, LA 70471
(504) 626-1985
FAX (504) 626-7029
compmedservices@home.com
CT,FP,NT,PM

METAIRIE

James P. Carter, MD, APCT
3501 Severn, #19
Metairie, LA 70002
(504) 779-6363
FAX (504) 779-9963
GP,NT,PM

Janet Perez-Chiesa, MD,
BPCT
4532 W. Napoleon Ave., #210
Metairie, LA 70001
(504) 456-7539
FAX (504) 456-7542
CT,GP,IM,PM, Neurology

Kashi Rai, MD, BPCT
4720 S. I-10 Service Rd., #305
Metairie, LA 70001
(504) 454-8952
FAX (504) 454-7708
A,CT,FP,HGL,NT,PM,GP

MAINE

GRAY

Raymond Psonak, DO
51 West Gray Rd., #1-A
P.O. Box 605
Gray, ME 04039-0605
(207) 657-4325
FAX (207) 657-4325
medinfo@healthallways.com
A,CT,DD,NT,Immune D/O,
Env. Med.

PORTLAND

Alan N. Weiner, DO
4 Milk Street
Portland, ME 04101
(207) 828-8080
FAX (207) 828-6816
Email: anw@webmail.une.edu
CT,NT,AC,OS,Anti-Aging,Env. Med.

MARYLAND

ANNAPOLIS

Richard A. Bernstein, MD
133 Defense Hwy., #109
The Courtyards
Annapolis, MD 21401
(410) 224-5558
FAX (410) 224-7321
A,IM,NT,PM,PUD,YS

Jacob E. Teitelbaum, MD
466 Forelands Road
Annapolis, MD 21401
(410) 573-5389
FAX (410) 266-6104
IM

BALTIMORE

Binyamin Rothstein, DO, APCT
2835 Smith Ave., #209
Baltimore, MD 21209
(410) 484-2121
A,CT,GP,NT,OS,RHU

BELCAMP

Philip W. Halstead, MD
1200 Brass Mill Road
Belcamp, MD 21017
(410) 272-7751
FAX (410) 273-0476
IM,DIA,NT,PM

BETHESDA

Norton Fishman, MD
5413 W. Cedar lane, #205-C
Bethesda, MD 20814
(301) 897-3599
FAX (301) 564-3116
CT,GER,IM,PM

Lillian Somner, DO
9213 Seven Locks Road
Bethesda, MD 20817
(301) 469-8900
FAX (301) 767-0695
P,OSM,AC

COLLEGE PARK

Floyd E. Taub, MD
387 Technology Dr., #2119
College Park, MD 20742
(301) 405-0743
FAX (301) 405-9187
Pathology, Immunology

EASTON

Paul V. Beals, MD, BPCT
Easton Plaza
101 Marlboro Rd., #25
Easton, MD 21601
(410) 770-5900
CT,FP,NT,PM

LAUREL

Paul V. Beals, MD, BPCT
9101 Cherry Lane Park, Suite
205
Laurel, MD 20708
(301) 490-9911
CT,FP,NT,PM

LUTHERVILLE

Elisabeth Lucas, MD
2328 W. Joppa Rd., #310
Lutherville, MD 21093
(410) 823-3101
FAX (410) 296-0650
Email: eklucas@juno.com
IM

Kenneth B. Singleton, MD
2328 W. Joppa Rd., #310
Lutherville, MD 21093
(410) 296-3737
FAX (410) 296-0650
IM,NT,AC

WALDORF

F. Alexander Leon, MD
85 High Street
Walforf, MD 20602
(301) 645-9551
FAX (301) 645-1009
FP,NT

MASSACHUSETTS

ARLINGTON

Michael Janson, MD, FACAM, APCT
180 Massachusetts Ave.
Arlington, MA 02474
(781) 641-1901
FAX (781) 641-3963
Email: drjanson@drjanson.com
A,CD,CT,NT,OME,YS

BOSTON

Ruben Oganesov, MD, APCT
39 Brighton Ave.
Boston, MA 02134
(617) 783-5783
FAX (617) 783-1519
AC,CT,GP,NT,PMR

Earl Robert Parson, MD
495 Summer Street (MEPS)
Boston, MA 02210
(617) 753-3113
Email: senior2020@aol.com
CT,AR,DD,GP,PM,WR

CAMBRIDGE

Leonid Gordin, MD
2500 Massachusetts Ave.
Cambridge, MA 02140
(617) 661-6225
FAX (617) 492-2002
AU,DD,CT,HGL,NT,YS

Guy Pugh, MD, BPCT
2500 Massachusetts Ave.
Cambridge, MA 02140
(617) 661-6225
FAX (617) 492-2002
A,AC,CT,GP,NT,IM

Vladimir P. Shurlan, MD
7 Channing St.
Cambridge, MA 02138
(617) 547-3249
FAX (617) 547-3249
DD,FP,IM,NT,PM,PMR,S

MALDEN

George Milowe, MD, APCT
11 Bickford Road
Maiden, MA 02148
(781) 397-7408
AC,CT,NT,PM,PO, Herbs

MANSFIELD

Marcia Lipski, MD
450 Chauncy Street
Mansfield, MA 02048
(508) 339-7788
FP

NEWTON

Carol Englender, MD, BPCT
1126 Beacon St.
Newton, MA 02461
(617) 965-7770
A,FP,NT,PM,Env. Med.

Jeanne Hubbuch, MD
1126 Beacon St.
Newton, MA 02461
(617) 965-7770
A,CT,FP,GYN,NT,YS

NORTHAMPTON

Barry D. Elson, MD
52 Maplewood Shops – Old South St.
Horthampton, MA 01060
(413) 584-7787
FAX (413) 584-7778
A,CT,NT,PM,YS

S. YARMOUTH

Paul Cochrane, DO
23G White's Path
S. Yarmouth, MA 02664
(508) 760-2423
FAX (508) 760-1019
AC,CT,FP,GP,OS,PM

WEST BOYLSTON

N. Thomas La Cava, MD
360 West Boylston St., Suite 107
West Boylston, MA 01583
(508) 854-1380
FAX (508) 854-1377
NT,PD,PM,CT,A,YS

MICHIGAN

BAY CITY

Parveen A. Malik, MD
808 N. Euclid Ave.
Bay City, MI 48706
(517) 686-3760
BA,CT,FP,GP,NT,PM

CLARKSTON

Nedra Downing, DO, BPCT
5639 Sashabaw Road
Clarkston, MI 48346
(248) 625-6677
FAX (248) 625-5633
A,GP,NT,OS,PM,YS

FLINT

William M. Bernard, DO, BPCT
1044 Gilbert Street
Flint, MI 48532
(810) 733-3140
FAX (810) 733-5623
A,CT,FP,GER,OSM,PM

Kenneth Ganapini, DO
1044 Gilbert Street
Flint, MI 48532
(810) 733-3140
FAX (810) 733-5623
Email: KGanap@aol.com
CT,FP,GP,OSM,PM,YS

Janice Shimoda, DO, BPCT
1044 Gilbert Street
Flint, MI 48532
(810) 733-3140
FAX (810) 733-5623
CT,FP,NT,PM

GRAND RAPIDS

Arden B. Andersen, DO, BPCT
3700 – 52nd Street S.E.
Grand Rapids, MI 49512
(616) 656-3700
FAX (616) 656-3701
CT,HO,NT,OS,PM,YS

Tammy Born, DO, APCT
3700 – 52nd Street S.E.
Grand Rapids, MI 49512
(616) 656-3700
FAX (616) 656-3701
Email: tborn@bornclinic.com
CT,GP,PM,YS,Laser

GROSSE POINTE

R.B. Fahim, MD, BPCT
20825 Mack Ave.
Grosse Pointe, MI 48236
(313) 640-9730
FAX (313) 640-9740
CT,MM

HUNTINGTON WOODS

Philip Hoekstra, III, PhD
26711 Woodward Ave., #203
Huntington Woods, MI 48070
HONORARY MEMBER

LAPEER

Paul D. Lepor, DO, BPCT
1254 North Main St.
Lapeer, MI 48446
(810) 664-4531
A,PD

MIDLAND

Bharti Jain, MD
212 W. Wackerly St. #B
Midland, MI 48640
(517) 837-5998
FAX (517) 835-9632
CT,FP,GP,NT,PM,PMR,YS

NORWAY

F. Michael Saigh, MD
411 Murray Rd. West U.S. 2
Norway, MI 49870
(906) 563-9600
FAX (906) 563-7110
FP

PARCHMENT

Eric Born, DO, APCT
2350 East G Avenue
Parchment, MI 49004
(616) 344-6183
FAX (616) 349-3046
DIA,FP,NT,OS,PM,YS

PONTIAC

Vahagn Agbabian, DO
28 No. Saginaw St., Suite 1105
Pontiac, MI 48342-2144
(248) 334-2424
FAX (248) 334-2924
CT,DD,DIA,GER,IM,OME

ROCKFORD

Robert A. DeJonge, DO, BPCT
350 Northland Drive
Rockford, MI 49341
(616) 866-4474
FAX (616) 866-4476
FP,Anti-Aging,NT

ROMEO

James Ziobron, DO
71441 Van Dyke
Romeo, MI 48065
(810) 336-3700
FAX (810) 336-9443
A,CT,DD,F,P,YS

SALINE

John G. Ghuneim, MD, BPCT
420 Russell, #204
Saline Prof. Office Bldg.
Saline, MI 48176
(734) 429-2581
FAX (734) 429-3410
AC,AU,CT,IM,NT,PM,P/S

TAWAS CITY

Michael D. Papenfuse, DO
200 Hemlock Rd.
Tawas City, MI 48764
(517) 362-9229
FAX (517) 362-9228
AN,OS,P/S,YS

WEST BLOOMFIELD

David Brownstein, MD
5821 W. Maple Rd., #192
West Bloomfield, MI 48322
(248) 851-1600
FAX (248) 851-0421
FP,AC,A

MINNESOTA

ALBERT LEA

Jean R. Eckerly, MD, APCT
216 E. Main Street
Albert Lea, MN 56007
(952) 593-9458
CT,IM,NT,OME,PM

MINNETONKA

Jean R. Eckerly, MD, APCT
13911 Ridgedale Dr., #350
Minnetonka, MN 55441
(952) 593-9458
FAX (952) 593-0097
CT,IM,NT,OME,PM

PAYNESVILLE

Tom Sult, MD, BPCT
200 First St. West
Paynesville, MN 56362
(320) 243-3767
GP

ST. LOUIS PARK

Michael A. Dole, MD, APCT
3408 Dakota So.
St. Louis Park, MN 55416
(612) 924-1053
FAX (612) 924-0254
CT,FP,PM,YS

ST. PETER

Harold J. Fletcher, MD
220 West Broadway
St. Peter, MN 56082
(507) 934-4850
FAX (507) 934-4909
CT,FP,GE,NT,P/S

MISSISSIPPI

COLDWATER

Pravin P. Patel, MD
P.O. Box 1060
Coldwater, MS 38618
(601) 622-7011
CT,FP

COLUMBUS

Jacob Skiwski, MD, BPCT
3491 Bluecutt Rd.
Columbus, MS 39701
(601) 329-2955 or 327-0646
A,CT,NT,GP,PD

OCEAN SPRINGS

James H. Waddell, MD
1520 Government Street
Ocean Springs, MS 39564
(228) 875-5505
AC,AN,AU,CT

MISSOURI

BRANSON

Brian Dieterie, MD
221 Skaggs Road, #102
Branson, MO 65616
(417) 334-0813
FAX (417) 334-6685

BRIDGETON

Harvey Walker Jr., MD, PhD,
FACAM, APCT
11995 Beaverton Dr.
Bridgeton, MO 63044
NO REFERRALS

FLORISSANT

Tipu Sultan, MD
11585 W. Florissant
Florissant, MO 63033
(314) 921-7100
A,AR,CT,HGL,PM

INDEPENDENCE

Lawrence Dorman, DO
9120 E. 35th Street
Independence, MO 64052
(816) 358-2712
AC,CT,MM,OSM,PM

JOPLIN

Ralph D. Cooper, DO, BPCT
1608 E. 20th Street
Joplin, MO 64804
(417) 624-4323
FP,GP,GYN,OS,S

SPRINGFIELD

Neil Nathan, MD
2828 N. National, #D
Springfield, MO 65803
(417) 869-7583
FAX (417) 869-7592
neilnathan@worldnet.att.net
AC,CT,FP,NT,OS,PM

William C. Sunderwirth,
DO, BPCT
2828 N. National
Springfield, MO 65803
(417) 837-4158
FAX (417) 837-4025
CT,DIA,GP,OSM,PM,S

ST. LOUIS

Lena R. Capapas, MD, BPCT
3009 N. Ballas Rd., #140-A
St. Louis, MO 63131
(314) 995-9713
FAX (314) 995-9818
IM,CD

Octavio R. Chirino, MD
9701 Landmark Pdwy. Dr., #207
St. Louis, MO 63127
(314) 842-4802
OBS,GYN,NT, Hormone Repl.

Varsha Rathod, MD
1977 Schueltz Rd.
St. Louis, MO 63146
(314) 997-5403
FAX (314) 997-6837
IM,CT,DIA,AR,NT, HGL,YS

Simon M. Yu, MD, APCT
11710 Old Ballas Rd., #205
St. Louis, MO 63141
(314) 432-7802
FAX (314) 432-1971
CD,CT,DIA,IM,NT,PM

MONTANA

BILLINGS

David C. Healow, MD
1242 North 28th, #1001
Billings, MT 59102
(406) 252-6674
AC,AN

BOZEMAN

Curt Kurtz, MD
300 N. Willson, #502E
Bozeman, MT 59715
(406) 587-5561
FAX (406) 585-8536
FP,HYP,YS

GREAT FALLS

Bonnie Friehling, MD
2517 7th Ave. South, #A-3
Great Falls, MT 59405
(406) 761-5778
FAX (406) 761-7117
Email: bfriehling@msn.com
GP,FP

ST. IGNATIUS

Mary Stranahan, DO
P.O. Box 430
St. Ignatius, MT 59865
(406) 745-3600
FAX (406) 745-4757
GP,NT,OS

WHITE SULPHUR
SPRINGS

Daniel J. Gebhardt, MD
Box 338 – 12 E. Main
White Sulphur Springs, MT 59645
(406) 547-3384
CT,GP,GYN,IM,PM,RHU

NEBRASKA

HARTINGTON

Steve Vlach, MD
405 W. Darlene St., P.O. Box 937
Hartington, NE 68739
(402) 254-3935
FAX (402) 254-2393
CD,CT,DIA,FP,NT,WR,YS,Emerg.
Med.

OMAHA

Eugene C. Oliveto, MD
10804 Prairie Hills Dr.
Omaha, NE 68144
(402) 392-0233
CT,HYP,NT,PM,P,PO

Jeffrey Passer, MD
9300 Underwood Ave., Suite 520
Omaha, NE 68114
(402) 398-1200
FAX (402) 398-9119
BA,CT,IM,PM

NEVADA

CARSON CITY

Frank Shallenberger, MD, HMD
896 W. Nye Lane, #103
Carson City, NV 89703
(775) 884-3990
FAX (775) 884-2202
CT,GP,HOM, Neurol, Ther, Oxid.
Med.

HENDERSON

Dan F. Royal, DO
2501 N. Green Valley Pkwy.,
#D-132
Henderson, N.W. 89014
(702) 443-8800
FAX (702) 433-8823
Email: royal@drroyal.com
A,CT,HYP,NT,OS,PM

LAS VEGAS

Steven Holper, MD
3233 W. Charleston, #202
Las Vegas, NV 89102
(702) 878-3510
FAX (702) 878-1405
Phys. Rehab.

Paul M. McHugh, DO
2250 E. Tropicana Ave., #19,
PMB 281
Las Vegas, NV 89119
(619) 543-9410
FAX (619) 543-0814
CT,FP,GP,OS

Robert D. Milne, MD
2110 Pinto Lane
Las Vegas, NV 89106
(702) 385-1393
FAX (702) 385-4170
Email: mmc@lvcm.com
A,AC,CT,FP,NT,PM

F. Fuller Royal, MD
3663 Pecos McLeod
Las Vegas, NV 89121
(702) 732-1400
FAX (702) 732-9661
A,AC,CT,GP,HYP

Robert Vance, DO, APCT
2746 Desert Zinnia Lane
Las Vegas, NV 89135-2000
HONORARY MEMBER

RENO

W. Douglas Brodie, MD, MD
(H)
601 West Moana Lane
Reno, NV 89509
(775) 829-1009
FAX (775) 829-9330
CT,DD,FP,GP,HOM,IM,NT,PM

David A. Edwards, MD, APCT
6490 S. McCarran Blvd., #C-24
Reno, NV 89509
(775) 827-1444
FAX (775) 827-2424
cora@bioregen.reno.nv.us
A,AC,CT,DD,PM,YS

Michael L. Gerber, MD, APCT
3670 Grant Dr., #101
Reno, NV 89509
(775) 826-1900
AC,CD,END,GP,HOM,NT,PD

Corazon Ibarra-Ilarina, MD,
MD (H), APCT
6490 S. McCarran Blvd., #C-24
Reno, NV 89509
(775) 827-1444
FAX (775) 827-2424
cora@bioregen.reno.nv.us
CT,PM, Biol. Med

NEW HAMPSHIRE

MANCHESTER

Judson R. Belmont, MD, BPCT
130 Tarrytown Rd.
Manchester, NH 03103
(603) 669-0831
jbelmont@cyberportal.net
A,CT,MM,NT,RHI,YS

NEW JERSEY

BERKELEY HEIGHTS

Daniel Zacharias, MD, BPCT
369 Springfield Ave.
Berkeley Heights, NJ 07922
(908) 464-6700
GP, Emerg. Med.

BLOOMFIELD

Majid Ali, MD
320 Belleville Ave.
Bloomfield, NJ 07003
(973) 586-4111
A,PM,Pathology

Richard L. Podkul, MD
1064 Broad Street
Bloomfield, NJ 07003
(973) 893-0282
FAX (973) 893-0612
CT,A,IM,NT,DIA

Raymond P. Russomanno, MD
350 Bloomfield Ave., #1
Bloomfield, NJ 07003
(973) 748-9330
IM

BRICK

Ivan Krohn, MD
1140 Burnt Tavern Road
Brick, NJ 08724
(732) 785-2670
FAX (732) 785-2673
CT,CD,DD,GP,PM,NT

BRIGANTINE

Michael J. Dunn, MD
4248 Harbor Beach Blvd.
Brigantine, NJ 08203
(609) 266-0400
FAX (609) 266-2597
IM,CT

CEDAR GROVE

Robert Steinfeld, MD
912 Pompton Ave., #9-B-1
Canfield Ofc.Pk.
Cedar Grove, NJ 07009
(973) 243-9898
FAX (973) 835-8312
CD,CT,DD,NT,PM,S

CHERRY HILL

Scott R. Greenberg, MD, BPCT
1907 Greentree Rd.
Cherry Hill, NJ 08003
(856) 424-8222
FAX (856) 424-2599
CT,P/S,FP,PM,MM,NT

Alan Magaziner, DO, FACAM, APCT
1907 Greentree Road
Cherry Hill, NJ 08003
(856) 424-8222
FAX (856) 424-2599
Email: amagaziner@aol.com
A,CT,DD,NT,OME,OSM,PM

DENVILLE

Majid Ali, MD
95 E. Main Street, #101
Denville, NJ 07834
(973) 586-4111
FAX (973) 586-8466
A,PM,Pathology

EDISON

Richard B. Menashe, DO
15 South Main St.
Edison, NJ 08837
(732) 906-8866
FAX (732) 906-0124
A,CD,CT,HGL,NT,YS

James Neubrander, MD
15 S. Main Street, #6
Edison, NJ 08837
(732) 634-3666
FAX (732) 634-8008
A,CT,MM,NT,PM,YS

ELIZABETH

Gennaro Locurcio, MD, BPCT
610 Third Avenue
Elizabeth, NJ 07202
(908) 351-1333
FAX (908) 351-3740
A,AC,CT,NT,P/S,PO

FAIR LAWN

Anthony M. Giliberti, DO
14-01 Broadway
Fair Lawn, NJ 07410
(201) 797-8534
GP,A,CD,DD,NT,PM

FORKED RIVER

Mark J. Bartiss, MD, BPCT
933 Lacey Road
Forked River, NJ 08050
(609) 693-2000
BA,CT,DD,FP,NT,PM

FORT LEE

Gary Klingsberg, DO, APCT
1355 15th Street, #200
Fort Lee, NJ 07024
(201) 585-9368
FAX (201) 585-0162
A,CT,Env.Med.,PM,YS

HACKENSACK

Robin Leder, MD, APCT
235 Prospect Ave.
Hackensack, NJ 07601
(201) 525-1155
A,CT,NT,PM

HADDONFIELD

Roberta Morgan, DO, BPCT
255 Kings Hwy. E.
Haddonfield, NJ 08033
(856) 216-9001
CT,GP,GYN,PM,NT,OSM

LAKEWOOD

Gloria Freundlich, DO
122 Hope Chapel Road
Lakewood, NJ 08701
(732) 961-9217
CT,FP,NT,OSM,PM

MANASQUAN

Vladimir Berkovich, MD, DC, BPCT
1707 Atlantic Ave., Bldg. B
Manasquan, NJ 08736
(732) 292-2101
FAX (732) 292-2105
CT,A,AC,NT,P/S,PM

MIDDLETOWN

David Dornfield, DO
18 Leonardville Rd.
Middletown, NJ 07748
(732) 671-3730
FAX (732) 706-1078
CT,DD,DIA,FP,NT,OSM,PM,PMR

Neil Rosen, DO
18 Leonardville Rd.
Middletown, NJ 07748
(732) 671-3730
FAX (732) 706-1078
FP,NT,OS,PM,PMR

MILLBURN

Sharda Sharma, MD
131 Millburn Avenue
Millburn, NJ 07041
(973) 376-4500
FAX (973) 467-2285
Email: sharmamd@aol.com
FP,AC,NT,CT

MORRIS PLAINS

Faina Munits, MD
39 East Hanover Avenue, Unit 3
Morris Plains, NJ 07950
(973) 292-3222
FAX (973) 292-3443
A,CD,CT,DIA,DD,HGL,PM

NORTH WILDWOOD

John G. Costino, DO
404 Surf Avenue
North Wildwood, NJ 08260
(609) 522-8358
FAX (609) 729-8662
GP,RHU,PMR,DD,FP, GER

NORTHFIELD

Barry D. Glasser, MD
1907 New Road
Northfield, NJ 08225
(609) 646-9600
FAX (609) 484-8127
AC,FP,IM,R,Pain Mngt.

PARAMUS

Thomas A. Cacciola, MD, BPCT
403 Farview Ave.
Paramus, NJ 07652
(201) 261-8386
FAX (201) 261-8827
CT,IM,NT,PM

RIDGEWOOD

Arie Rave, MD, BPCT
1250 E. Ridgewood Ave.
Ridgewood, NJ 07450
(201) 689-1900
FAX (201) 447-9011
CD,CT,FP,HGL,IM,NT,RHU

Stuart Weg, MD, BPCT
1250 E. Ridgewood Ave.
Ridgewood, NJ 07450
(201) 447-5558
FAX (201) 447-9011
AN,CT,DD,Pain Mngt.

SHREWSBURY

David Dornfield, DO
167 Avenue at the Commons, #1
Shrewsbury, NJ 07702
(732) 389-6455
FAX (732) 389-6365
CT,DD,DIA,FP,NTOSM,PM,PMR

Neil Rosen, DO
555 Shrewsbury Ave.
Shrewsbury, NJ 07702
(732) 219-0894
FAX (732) 219-0895
FP,NT,OS,PM,PMR

SOMERSET

Marc Condren, MD
15 Cedar Grove Lane, #20
Somerset, NJ 08873
(908) 469-2133
A,FP,MM,NT

STOCKTON

Stuart H. Freednenfeld, MD
56 So. Main St., #A
Stockton, NJ 08559
(609) 397-8585
FAX (609) 397-9335
A,AC,CT,END,FP,GYN

TRENTON

Imtiaz Ahmad, MD
1760 Whitehorse Hamilton Sq.
Rd. #5
Trenton, NJ 08690
(609) 890-2966
FAX (609) 890-3326
CD,S

Robert J. Peterson, DO
2239 Whitehorse/ Mercerville
Rd., #4
Trenton, NJ 08619
(215) 579-0330
AR,CD,CT,DD,DIA,NT,PM,YS

UNION CITY

Michael J. Calache, MD
4418 Kennedy Blvd.
Union City, NJ 07087
(201) 863-3111
IM,CT,NT,PM,DIA, HGL

WOODBRIDGE

David M. Strassberg, MD
1 Woodbridge Ctr., #245
Woodbridge, NJ 07095
(732) 855-7700
GE,IM,NT,CD,CT,DIA

NEW MEXICO

ALBUQUERQUE

Ralph J. Luciani, DO, APCT
10601 Lomas Blvd. N.E., #103
Albuquerque, NM 87112
(505) 298-5995
FAX (505) 298-2940
AC,AU,CT,FP,OSM,PM

Joseph P. Walter, MD
3415 Carlisle N.E.
Albuquerque, NM 87110
(505) 271-4800
FAX (505) 271-4882
A,CT,GP,GYN,NT,PM

LAS CRUCES

Burton M. Berkson, MD, PhD
741 N. Alameda, #12
Las Cruces, NM 88005
(505) 524-3720
FAX (505) 521-1815
Integrative Medicine

SANTA FE

Shirley B. Scott, MD
P.O. Box 2670
Santa Fe, NM 87504
(505) 986-9960
GE,MM,PM,YS

W. A. Shrader, Jr., MD
2422 Camino de Vida
Santa Fe, NM 87505
(505) 983-8890
FAX (505) 820-7315
shrader2@ix.netcom.com
A,NT,Env.Med.

NEW YORK

ALBANY

Kenneth A. Bock, MD,
FACAM, APCT
10 McKown Rd.
Pinnacle Place, Suite 210
Albany, NY 12203
(518) 435-0082
FAX (518) 435-0086
A,CD,CT,FP,NT,PM

ALBERTSON

Steven Rachlin, MD
927 Willis Avenue
Albertson, L.I., NY 11507
(516) 873-7773
FAX (516) 877-7365
A,CT,IM,NT,PM

BREWSTER

Jeffrey C. Kopelson, MD
221 Clock Tower Commons
Brewster, NY 10509
(914) 278-6800
FAX (914) 278-6897
CT,FP,NT,PM

Neil C. Raff, MD
192 Route 22, Suite 100
Brewster, NY 10509
(914) 277-7900
FAX (914) 277-7905
IM,GE

BRONX

David Dayya, DO
3rd Avenue and 183rd Street
Bronx, NY 10457
NO REFERRALS

Richard Izquierdo, MD, BPCT
1070 Southern Blvd., Lower
Level
Bronx, NY 10459
(718) 589-4541
A,FP,GP,NT,PD,PM

BRONXVILLE

Joseph S. Wojcik, MD
525 Bronxville Rd., 1-G
Bronxville, NY 10708
(914) 793-6161
A,CT,PD,PM,NT, Env. Med.

BROOKLYN

Gloria W. Freundlich, DO
575 Ocean Parkway
Brooklyn, NY 11218
(718) 437-4459
CT,FP,NT,OSM,PM

Levi H. Lehv, MD
6910 Avenue
Brooklyn, NY 11234
(718) 251-1200
BA,CT,DIA,IM,PM, HOM

Igor Ostrovsky, MD
3120 Brighton 5th Street, #1-C
Brooklyn, NY 11235
(718) 934-1920
FAX (718) 934-2078
AN,AC,CT,NT

Michael Teplitsky, MD
415 Oceanview Ave.
Brooklyn, NY 11235
(718) 769-0997
FAX (718) 646-2352
A,CD,CT,DIA,IM,PM

Pavel Yutsis, MD, APCT
6413 Bay Parkway
Brooklyn, NY 11204
(718) 621-0900
FAX (718) 621-9165
A,CT,FP,NT,PD,PM,YS

BUFFALO

Kalpana Patel, MD, APCT
65 Wehrle Drive
Buffalo, NY 14225
(716) 833-2213
FAX (716) 833-2244
A,CT,NT,PD,PM,HGL, YS

CHAPPAQUA

Savely Yurkovsky, MD
37 King Street
Chappaqua, NY 10514
(516) 333-2929
A,CD,CS,CT,NT,PM

EAST MEADOW

Kathryn Calabria, DO, BPCT
30 Merrick Ave., #110
East Meadow, NY 11554
(376) 542-9090
FAX (376) 542-9258
kecalabria@earthlink.net
AC,FP,OSM

EAST NORWICH

John B. Caramagna, DO, BPCT
73 Floyd Place
East Norwich, NY 11732
(516) 922-2157
FAX (516) 922-2158
Email: jcara@optonline.net
FP,OS,PM,PMR,NT,CT

FREDONIA

Robert F. Barnes, DO, BPCT
3489 E. Main Rd.
Fredonia, NY 14063
(716) 679-3510
FAX (716) 679-3512
Email: doctorrbarnes@aol.com
CT,NT,PM

GLENS FALLS

Ann Auburn, DO
15 W. Notre Dame Street
Glens Falls, NY 12801
(518) 745-7473
FAX (518) 792-7310
Email: aauburn@capital.net
CT,NT,PM,A,P/S,OSM

Andrew W. Garner, MD
8 Harrison Avenue
Glens Falls, NY 12801
(518) 798-9401
FAX (518) 798-9411
FP,CT,PM

GREAT NECK

Mary F. Di Rico, MD
1 Kingspoint Rd.
Great Neck, NY 11024
NO REFERRALS

HAMBURG

Robert F. Barnes, DO, BPCT
5225 Southwestern Blvd.
Hamburg, NY 14075
(716) 649-0225
FAX (716) 649-0369
CT,NT,PM

Ronald P. Santasiero, MD
5451 Southwestern Blvd.
Hamburg, NY 14075
(716) 646-6075
FAX (716) 646-5912
AC,CT,PM,P/S

LAKE SUCCESS

Maurice Cohen, MD
2 ProHealth Plaza
Lake Success, NY 11042
(516) 608-2806
FAX (516) 608-2805
mcohen@prohealthcare.com
GYN

LAWRENCE

Mitchell Kurk, MD, APCT
310 Broadway
Lawrence, NY 11559
(516) 239-5540
FAX (516) 371-2919
CT,FP,GER,NT,OME,PM

LEWISTON

Donald M. Fraser, MD
5147 Lewiston Rd.
Lewiston, NY 14092
(716) 284-5777
Orth.Surg.

MAMARONECK

Monica Furlong, MD
921 W. Boston Post Rd.
Mamaroneck, NY 10543
(914) 381-7687
FAX (914) 381-0942
AC,AN,CT,NT,Pain Mgmt., Neural
Therapy

MERRICK

Susan Groh, MD
2916 Frankel Blvd.
Merrick, NY 11566
(516) 867-5132
FAX (516) 867-5519
CT,FP,GER

MIDDLETOWN

Levi H. Lehv, MD
825 Route 211 East
Middletown, NY 10941
(914) 692-8338
FAX (914) 692-6177
BA,CT,DIA,IM,PM,HOM

NEW CITY

Arthur Landau, MD, BPCT
10 Esquire Road
New City, NY 10956
(914) 638-4464
FAX (914) 638-4509
A,BA,CT,IM,PM

NEW ROCHELLE

Harold C. Clark, MD
400 Webster Ave.
New Rochelle, NY 10801
(914) 235-8385
CT,DIA,GP,IM,NT,YS

NEW YORK

Richard N. Ash, MD
800-A Fifth Ave. 61st St.
New York, NY 10021
(212) 758-3200
FAX (212) 754-5800
Email: dr.ash@ashcenter.com
A,CD,CT,HYP,NT,MM,IM, Rec.
Therapy

Robert C. Atkins, MD
152 E. 55th St.
New York, NY 10022
(212) 758-2110
FAX (212) 751-1863
CT,HGL,OME

Eric R. Braveman, MD, APCT
185 Madison Ave., 6th floor
New York, NY 10016-4325
(212) 213-6155
FAX (212) 213-6188
CT,IM,MM,PM,PO, Neurology

Richard P. Brown, MD
30 East End Avenue, #1B
New York, NY 10028
(212) 737-0821
FAX (914) 331-3562
GP

Claudia M. Cooke, MD
133 East 73rd Street, #506
New York, NY 10021
(212) 861-9000
FAX (212) 585-4177
AC,IM,PM,NT

Ronald Hoffman, MD,
FACAM, APCT
40 E. 30th Street
New York, NY 10016
(212) 779-1744
FAX (212) 779-0891
Email: drrhoffman@aol.com
A,FP,HGL,NT,PM

Warren Levin, MD, APCT
31 East 28th Street, 6th Flr.
New York, NY 10016
(212) 679-9667
FAX (212) 679-9730
A,AC,CT,NT,OME,PM

Gennaro Locurcio, MD, BPCT
112 Lexington Avenue
New York, NY 10016
(212) 696-2680
FAX (212) 696-2694
A,AC,CT,NT,P/S,PO

Fred Pescatore, MD, BPCT
333 East 57th St., #1-B
New York, NY 10022
(212) 751-2318
FAX (212) 223-9757
CT,DIA,END,GP,PM,PH

Stephen D. Siegel, MD
3 East 71st Street at Fifth Avenue
New York, NY 10021
(212) 879-8000
FAX (212) 2888-5961
PUD,IM,GER,A

Francesca Skolas, MD, BPCT
200 Park Ave. South, 3rd Floor
New York, NY 10003
(212) 780-4459
FAX (212) 420-7211
FP,NT,PM

Michael J. Teplitsky, MD
31 East 28 Street
New York, NY 10016
(212) 679-3700
FAX (212) 679-9730
A,CD,CT,DIA,IM,PM

Lawrence Young, MD
19 Bowery Street, Rm. 1
New York, NY 10002-6702
(212) 431-4343
FAX (212) 925-8637
A,AC,NT,IM

NIAGARA FALLS

Paul Culter, MD, FACAM, APCT
652 Elmwood Ave.
Niagara Falls, NY 14301
(716) 284-5140
FAX (716) 284-5159
A,CT,NT

NO. WOODMERE

Bernard Lanter, MD, BPCT
461 Golf Court
No. Woodmere, NY 11581
(516) 763-2055
FAX (516) 766-3240
S,Alternative Medicine

ONEONTA

Richard Ucci, MD, APCT
521 Main Street
Oneonta, NY 13820
(607) 432-8752
CT,FP

ORANGEBURG

Neil L. Block, MD
14 Prel Plaza
Orangeburg, NY 10962
(914) 359-3300
A,CD,FP,IM,NT,PO

RHINEBECK

Kenneth A. Bock, MD,
FACAM, APCT
108 Montgomery St.
Rhinebeck, NY 12572
(845) 876-7082
FAX (845) 876-4615
A,CD,CT,FP,NT,PM

Steven Bock, MD
108 Montgomery Street
Rhinebeck, NY 12572
(845) 876-7082
FAX (845) 876-4615
bock@rhinebeckhealth.com
NT,CT,AC

SUFFERN

Michael B. Schachter, MD, FACAM, APCT
Two Executive Blvd., #202
Suffern, NY 10901
(914) 368-4700
FAX (914) 368-4727
mbschachter@mbschachter.com
A,CT,NT,PO

UTICA

Richard O'Brien, DO
2305 Genesee Street
Utica, NY 13501
(315) 724-8888
FP,CT,OM

Margarita Schilling, MD
2305 Genesee Street
Utica, NY 13501
(315) 797-3799
FAX (315) 734-1912
Email: mschil4455@aol.com
IM,END

WESTBURY

Savely Yurkovsky, MD
309 Madison St.
Westbury, NY 11590
(516) 333-2929
A,CD,CS,CT,NT,PM

WOODSIDE

Fira Nihamin, MD
39 – 65 52nd Street
Woodside, NY 11377
(718) 429-0039
FAX (718) 429-6965
CD,DIA,DD,GP,GER,IM

NORTH CAROLINA

ASHEVILLE

James Biddle, MD, APCT
239 S. French Broad Ave.
Asheville, NC 28801
(828) 252-5545
FAX (828) 281-3055
CT,CD,IM,NT,DIA

Ronald Parks, MD
20 Spring Hollow Circle
Asheville, NC 28805
(828) 298-7368
Integr.Med.,Env.Med., PO

John L. Wilson Jr., MD, APCT
Park Terrace Center,
1312 Patton Ave.
Asheville, NC 28806
(828) 252-9833
FAX (828) 255-8118
A,CT,Env.Med.,NT,PM

Eileen M. Wright, MD
Park Terrace Center,
1312 Patton Ave.
Asheville, NC 28806
(828) 252-9833
FAX (828) 255-8118
GP,PM

BANNER ELK

Charles Wiley, MD
64 High Country Square
Banner Elk, NC 28604
(828) 898-6949
FAX (828) 898-6950
A,AR,CT,FP,NT,PM,YS

CAROLINA BEACH

Keith E. Johnson, MD
1009 N. Lake Park Blvd., Box 16, C-5
Pleasure Island Plaza
Carolina Beach, NC 28428
(910) 458-0606
CD,CT,DIA,NT,PM,RHU,WR

CHARLOTTE

Rashid Ali Buttar, DO, APCT, FACAM
20721 Torrence Chapel, #101
Charlotte, NC 28031
(704) 895-9355
FAX (704) 895-9357
A,BA,CT,NT,PM,MM

Mark O'Neal Speight, MD, BPCT
2317 Randolph Rd.
Charlotte, NC 28207
(704) 334-8447
FAX (704) 334-0733
YS,CT,DD,RHU,NT,PO, MM

FLETCHER (ASHEVILLE)

Stephen Blievernicht, MD, BPCT
242 Old Concord Rd.
Fletcher (Asheville), NC 28732
(828) 684-4411
FAX (828) 684-7657
Email: drswb@mindspring.com
P/S,AC,AR,CD,CT,DD,DIA,MM

HILLSBOROUGH

Dennis W. Fera, MD, BPCT
1000 Corporate Dr., #209
Hillsborough (Chapel Hill), NC 27278
(919) 732-2287
FAX (919) 732-3176
CT,PM,NT,GP,OS,P/S

JACKSONVILLE

Subu Dubey, MD
25 Office Park Dr.
Jacksonville, NC 28546
(910) 355-2323
FAX (910) 355-0771
CS,CT,DIA,END,HO,IM,P

David Sheridad, MD
3220 Henderson Dr.
Jacksonville, NC 28546
(910) 938-9088
FAX (910) 938-3835
Email: dsheridan@ecorro.com
GP,CT

LAKE TOXAWAY

Richard Worsham, MD –
RETIRED
Route #1, Box #327-A
Lake Toxaway, NC 28747-9749
NO REFERRALS

MATTHEWS

Clarence E. Norris, MD, BPCT
13024-F Idlewild Road
Matthews, NC 28105
(704) 846-6071
FAX (704) 846-4800
AU,CT,FP,PMR

MONROE

Boyd W. Springs, MD
806 Circle Drive
Monroe, NC 28112
(704) 283-8626
FAX (704) 289-8212
GP,OBS

MOORESVILLE

Anthony J. Castiglia, MD,
BPCT
570 Williamson Road, Suite C
Mooresville, NC 28117
(704) 799-9740
FAX (704) 799-9742
FP,CT,AR,END,MM,NT,PM

MOREHEAD CITY

Donald Brooks Reece II,
MD, BPCT
#2 Medical Park
Morehead City, NC 28557
(252) 247-5177
FAX (252) 247-0223
CT,FP,GER,P/S,PM,WR

MURPHY

Robert E. Moreland, MD
75 Medical Park Lance, #C
Murphy, NC 28906
(828) 837-7997
FP

RALEIGH

John C. Pittman, MD, APCT
4505 Fair Meadow Lane, #111
Raleigh, NC 27607
(919) 571-4391
FAX (919) 571-8968
Email: info@carolinacenter.com
CT,GP,END,NT,PM,YS

Thomas Spruill, MD
3900 Browning Place, #201
Raleigh, NC 27609
(919) 787-7125
FAX (919) 787-9952
Email: trspl@concentric.net
P,PO

ROANOKE RAPIDS

Bhaskar D. Power, MD
1201 E. Littleton Rd.
Roanoke Rapids, NC 27870
(252) 535-1412
Email: bpower@pol.net
A,AR,CT,DD,GP,HOM,NT,PM,PUD,
S

SOUTHERN PINES

Keith E. Johnson, MD
1852 U.S. Hwy. 1 South
Southern Pines, NC 28387
(910) 695-0335
FAX (910) 695-3697
CD,CT,DIA,NT,PM,RHU,WR

TRYON

Mack Stuart Bonner Jr.,
MD, BPCT
590 South Trade Street
Tryon, NC 28782
(828) 859-0420
FAX (828) 859-0422
CT,PM,NT,Emerg. Med.

Connie G. Ross, MD, BPCT
590 South Trade Street
Tryon, NC 28782
(828) 859-0420
FAX (828) 859-0422
CT,NT,PM

WINSTON-SALEM

Walter Ward, MD
1411B Plaza West Road
Winston-Salem, NC 27103
(336) 760-0240
FAX (336) 760-4568
A,CT,ENT,NT,RHI,YS

Laurence Webster, MD
2803 Lyndhurst Ave.
Winston-Salem, NC 27103
(336) 499-3800
A,CT,DD,NT,PM,YS, WR

NORTH DAKOTA
GRAND FORKS

Richard H. Leigh, MD, APCT
2600 Demers Ave., #108
Grand Forks, ND 58201
(701) 772-7696
FP

MINOT

Brian E. Briggs, MD
718 – 6th Street S.W.
Minot, ND 58701
(701) 838-6011
FAX (701) 838-5055
CT,FP,NT

OHIO
AKRON

Josephine C. Aronica, MD
1867 W. Market St.
Akron, OH 44313
(330) 867-7361
FAX (330) 867-7362
AC,CT,NT

BLUFFTON

L. Terry Chappell, MD,
FACAM, APCT
122 Thurman St. – Box 248
Bluffton, OH 45817
(419) 358-4627
FAX (419) 358-1855
Email: chappell@wcoil.com
AU,CT,FP,HYP,NT,PMR

CINCINNATI

Kaushal K. Bhardwaj, MD
9019 Colerain Ave.
Cincinnati, OH 45251
(513) 385-8100
FAX (513) 385-8106
A,AC,CT,IM, Prolotherapy

Ted Cole, DO, MA
9678 Cincinnati-Columbus Road
Cincinnati, OH 45241
(513) 779-0300
A,CT,FP,NT,OSM,PD

Leonid Macheret, MD
375 Glensprings Dr., #400
Cincinnati, OH 45246
(513) 851-8790
FAX (513) 851-0434
CT,GP,NT,PM

James E. Smith, DO, BPCT
11263 Reading Road
Cincinnati, OH 45241
(513) 769-7546
FAX (513) 769-7547
CD,CT,FP,NT,OSM,WR,YS

CLEVELAND

Radha Baishnab, MD
7215 Old Oak Blvd., #A-316
Cleveland, OH 44130
(440) 234-8080
FAX (440) 234-0525
CD,CT,IM,NT,PM

John M. Baron, DO, APCT
4807 Rockside, Suite 100
Cleveland, OH 44131
(216) 642-0082
FAX (216) 642-1415
CD,CT,MM,NT,PM, RHU

Ronald B. Casselberry, MD
2132 W. 25th Street
Cleveland, OH 44113
(216) 771-5855
FAX (216) 771-4534
AC,CT,DD,NT,OS,PM

James P. Frackelton, MD,
FACAM, APCT
24700 Center Ridge Rd.
Cleveland, OH 44145
(440) 835-0104
FAX (440) 871-1404
CT,HO,NT,PM

Stan Gardner, MD
24700 Center Ridge Rd.
Cleveland, OH 44145
(440) 835-0104
FAX (440) 871-1404
PM,PD,CT

Sakoo Lee, MD, BPCT
24700 Center Ridge Rd. #317
Cleveland, OH 44145
(440) 835-0104
FAX (440) 871-1404
FP,CT,PM,MM,HO

Derrick Lonsdale, MD,
FACAM, APCT
24700 Center Ridge Rd.
Cleveland, OH 44145
(440) 835-0104
FAX (440) 871-1404
Email: dlonsdale@pol.net
NT,PM,PD

COLUMBUS

Larry S. Everhart, MD
4825 Knights Bridge Blvd.
Columbus, OH 43214
(614) 326-2600
FAX (614) 326-2644
CD,DIA,IM,CT,NT

Bruce A. Massau, DO
1492 E. Broad St., #1203
Columbus, OH 43205-1546
(614) 252-1500
FAX (614) 252-1685
CT,Pain Mgmt.

LANCASTER

Jacqueline S. Chan, DO
3484 Cincinnati Zanesville Rd.
Lancaster, OH 43130
(740) 653-0017
FAX (740) 653-8707
CT,FP,OS,YS, Homeopathy

MANSFIELD

Ho Young Chung, MD, BPCT
812 Park Avenue East
Mansfield, OH 44905
(419) 589-8819
FAX (419) 589-8820
AN

PAULDING

Don K. Snyder, MD
1030 West Wayne Street
Paulding, OH 45879
(419) 399-2045
CT,FP

POWELL

William D. Mitchell, DO,
APCT
Entrance A, Suite 10
10401 Sawmill Pkwy.
Powell, OH 43065
(614) 761-0555
FAX (614) 761-8937
Email: drwdm@ix.netcom.com
CD,CT,GP,IM,PM,OSM

RICHMOND HEIGHTS

Ronald B. Casselberry, MD
27155 Chardon Road
Richmond Heights, OH 44143
(216) 771-5855
FAX (216) 771-4534
AC,CT,DD,NT,OS,PM

SANDUSKY

Douglas Weeks, MD, APCT
3703 Columbus Avenue
Sandusky, OH 44870
(419) 625-8085
CT,HO,NT,PM,AC,PMR

TOLEDO

James C. Roberts Jr., MD
4607 Sylvania Ave. #200
Toledo, OH 43623
(419) 882-9625
FAX (412) 882-9628
CD,IM,PM,EECP

VERSAILLES

Charles W. Platt, MD
552 South West Street
Versailles, OH 45380
(513) 526-3271
FAX (513) 526-5240
A,CT,FP,GP

YOUNGSTOWN

James Ventresco Jr., DO
3848 Tippecanoe Rd.
Youngstown, OH 44511
(330) 792-2349
CT,FP,NT,OSM,RHU

OKLAHOMA

JENKS

Gerald Wootan, DO, BPCT
715 West Main St., #S
Jenks, OK 74037
(918) 299-9447
FP,GER,OS,PD,A,GYN

OKLAHOMA CITY

Adam Merchant, MD
3535 N.W. 58th Street
Oklahoma City, OK 73112
(405) 942-8346
FAX (405) 942-8347
P/S,NT,AU,CT,AC

Charles D. Taylor, MD, APCT
4409 Classen Blvd.
Oklahoma City, OK 73118
(405) 525-7751
FAX (405) 525-0303
GP,GYN,OBS,PM,PMR

Ray E. Zimmer, DO
5419 S. Western Ave.
Oklahoma City, OK 73109
(405) 634-7855
FAX (405) 634-0778
A,CT,PM,RHU,DIA, OSM

PAWNEE

Gordon P. Laird, DO, BPCT
304 Boulder
Pawnee, OK 74058
(918) 762-3601
FAX (918) 762-2544
CT,GE,FP,PM,S

TULSA

R. Jeff Wright, DO
2488 E. 81st Street, Suite 485
Tulsa, OK 74137
(918) 496-5444
FAX (918) 496-5445
jeff.wright@ctcoftulsa.com
FP,OSM

VALLIANT

Ray E. Zimmer, DO
602 No. Dalton
Valliant, OK 74764
(580) 933-4235
A,CT,PM,RHU,DIA, OSM

OREGON

ASHLAND

Ronald Kapp, MD, PhD
P.O. Box 970
Ashland, OR 97520
NO REFERRALS

Franklin H. Ross Jr., MD
565 A Street
Ashland, OR 97520
(541) 482-7007
FAX (541) 482-5123
CT,DD,GP,GYN,NT,PM

EUGENE

John Gambee, MD
66 Club Road, #140
Eugene, OR 97401
(541) 686-2531
FAX (541) 686-2349
Email: jgambee@msn.com
A,CT,NT,PM,P/S

GRANTS PASS

James Fitzsimmons Jr., MD
591 Hidden Valley Rd.
Grants Pass, OR 97527
(541) 474-2166
A,CT

KLAMATH FALLS

Robert P. Beaman, MD
1903 Austin St., #B
Klamath Falls, OR 97603
(541) 885-9989
FAX (541) 885-7998
FP,CD,DIA,IM,PD,P

MEDFORD

Helen Trew, MD
2921 Doctor's Park Drive
Medford, OR 97504
(541) 770-1143
FAX (541) 772-9149
CT,FP,PM,Anti-Aging Med.

OREGON CITY

Jay A. Mead, MD
516 High Street
Oregon City, OR 97045
(503) 665-1644
FAX (503) 655-1720
CD,CT,DIA,END,MM,NT

PORTLAND

Richard C. Heitsch, MD
177 N.E. 102nd Avenue
Professional Plaza 102 Bldg. V
Portland, OR 97220
(503) 261-0966
FAX (503) 252-2691
A,CT,FP,GP,HGL,NT

Jeffrey Tyler, MD
163 N.E. 102nd Ave.
Portland, OR 97220
(503) 255-4256
CT,IM,GER,PD,PM

SALEM

Terence Howe Young, MD
1205 Wallace Rd. N.W.
Salem, OR 97304
(503) 371-1588
A,CT,GP,OSM,PM

SPRINGFIELD

Kathy Hirtz, MD
1800 Centennial Blvd., #6
Springfield, OR 97477
(541) 726-1865
FAX (541) 726-2179
BA,GP,PM

SWEET HOME

David J. Ogle, MD
2242 Main Street
Sweet Home, OR 97386
(541) 367-6137
FAX (541) 367-4114
FP

PENNSYLVANIA

BANGOR

Francis J. Cinelli, DO
153 N. 11th Street
Bangor, PA 18013
(610) 588-4502
FAX (610) 588-6928
CT,GP,HYP

BEDFORD

Ruth D. Jones, DO
342 S. Richard St.
Bedord, PA 15522
(814) 623-8414
CT,FP,NT,OSM,PM

BENSALEM

Robert J. Peterson, DO
2169 Galloway Rd.
Bensalem, PA 19020
(215) 579-0330
AR,CD,CT,DD,DIA,NT,PM,YS

BETHLEHEM

Sally Ann Rex, DO
1343 Easton Ave.
Bethlehem, PA 18018
(610) 866-0900
FAX (610) 866-8333
CT,GP,OS,PM,Occ.Med.

BREINIGSVILLE

Erik Von Kiel, DO, APCT
9331 West Hamilton Blvd.
Breinigsville, PA 18031
(610) 398-8310
FAX (610) 398-8313
A,BA,CT,FP,MM,NT

DARBY

Lance Wright, MD
112 S. 4th Street
Darby, PA 19023
(610) 461-6225
FAX (610) 583-3356
DD,HYP,NT,PM,PO, Integr.Med.

ERIE

Karl J. Falk, DO
4234 Buffalo Rd.
Erie, PA 16510
(814) 899-7777
FAX (814) 899-1945
CT,GP,PM,NT

FARRELL

Robert D. Multari, DO
2120 Likens Lane, #101
Farrell, PA 16121
(412) 981-3731
FAX (412) 981-3740
A,CD,DD,DIA,GE,IM

FOUNTAINVILLE

Harold H. Byer, MD, PhD, APCT
5045 Swamp Rd., #A-101
Fountainville, PA 18923
(215) 348-0443
FAX (215) 348-9124
AR,CT,DIA,S

GETTYSBURG

Iftikhar J. Mehdi, MD
555 McGlaughlin Rd.
Gettysburg, PA 17325
(717) 642-4269
FAX (717) 642-9348
GP,FP,EM

GREENSBURG

Ralph A. Miranda, MD,
FACAM, APCT
RD. #12 – Box 108
Greensburg, PA 15601
(724) 838-7632
FAX (724) 836-3655
CT,FP,NT,OME,PM

GREENVILLE

Roy E. Kerry, MD
17 Sixth Avenue
Greenville, PA 16125
(412) 588-2600
FAX (412) 588-6427
A,DD,EM,NT,OTO,YS

HAVERFORD

Conrad G. Maulfair, Jr., DO,
FACAM, APC
600 Haverford Rd., #200
Haverford, PA 19041
(610) 658-0220 or
(800) 733-4065
coleenmaulfair@enter.net
A,CT,HGL

HERSHEY

Adrian J. Hohenwarter, MD
326 W. Chocolate Ave.
Hershey, PA 17033
(717) 534-2481
FAX (717) 533-2442
CT,FP,GP,PM,Natural Horm. Repl.

JEANNETTE

R. Christopher Monsour, MD
70 Lincoln Way East
Monsour Medical Center
Jeannette, PA 15644
(412) 527-1511
Addiction, P

JEFFERSONVILLE

Anthony J. Bazzan, MD, BPCT
2505 Blvd. Of Generals
Jeffersonville, PA 19403
(610) 630-8600
FAX (610) 630-9599
Email: fwsi@msn.com
A,AC,CD,CT,DD,IM,YS

KENNETT SQUARE

Nicholas J. D'Orazio, MD
New Garden Plaza
747 W. Cypress St.
Kennett Square, PA 19348
(610) 444-1424
BA,CD,CT,DD,FP,NT

LEWISBURG

George C. Miller II, MD
3 Hospital Drive
Lewisburg, PA 17837
(717) 524-4405
FAX (717) 523-8844
GYN,OBS,YS

LOWER BURRELL

Lous K. Hauber, MD, BPCT
2533 Leechburg Rd.
Lower Burrell, PA 15680
(724) 334-0966
FAX (724) 339-4223
Email: MNIedta@Yahoo.com
CT,P,NT,Complimentary Medicine

MECHANICSBURG

Jeffrey A. Morrison, MD
1001 S. Market St.
Mechanicsburg, PA 17055
(717) 697-5050
FAX (717) 697-3156
A,CT,FP,NT,PM,YS

John M. Sullivan, MD, APCT
1001 S. Market St. #B
Merchanicsburg, PA 17055
(717) 697-5050
FAX (717) 697-3156
A,CT,DIA,FP,PD,YS

MEDIA

Arthur K. Balin, MD, PhD
110 Chesley Drive
Media, PA 19063
(610) 565-3300
FAX (610) 565-9909
CT,DD,END,GER,IM

MT. PLEASANT

Mamduh El-Attrache, MD
20 E. Main St.
Mt. Pleasant, PA 15666
(412) 547-3576
BA,CT,DIA,GER,OBS, PO

NARBERTH

Andrew Lipton, DO, APCT
822 Montgomery Ave. #315
Narberth, PA 19072
(610) 667-4601
FAX (610) 667-6416
Email: ALiptonDO@aol.com
CT,FP,OSM,AC

NEWTOWN

Robert J. Peterson, DO
1614 Wrightstown Rd.
Newtown, PA 18940
(215) 579-0330
AR,CD,CT,DD,DIA,NT,PM,YS

NORTH WALES

Domenick Braccia, DO, BPCT
1146 Stump Road
North Wales, PA 19454
(215) 368-2160
AC,FP,OS

PAOLI

Martin Mulders, MD
18 Paoli Pike, 1st Floor
Paoli, PA 19301
(610) 725-9996
FAX (610) 725-9997
CT,GP,IM,NT,PM

PENNDEL

Eric R. Braverman, MD, APCT
142 Bellevue Ave.
Penndel, PA 19047
(215) 702-1344
FAX (215) 757-1707
CT,IM,MM,PM,PO, Neurology

George Danielewski, MD
142 Bellevue Ave.
Penndel, PA 19047
(215) 757-4455
GP

PHILADELPHIA

George Danielewski, MD
7927 Fairfield St.
Philadelphia, PA 19152
(215) 338-8866
CD,CT,FP,GER,NT,PM

Sarah M. Fisher, MD, BPCT
530 South 2nd St., #108
Philadelphia, PA 19147
(215) 627-3001
FAX (215) 627-0362
GP,NT,YS,HOM

Alan F. Kwon, MD
211 South Street, #345
Philadelphia, PA 19147
(215) 629-5633
FAX (215) 629-5633
AN,HYP,PM,P/S,S

Patrick J. Lariccia, MD
51 N. 39th Street
Philadelphia, PA 19104-2640
(215) 662-8988
FAX (215) 662-8859
AC,HYP,PMR,YS

PITTSBURGH

Dominic A. Brandy, MD
2275 Swallow Hill Road, #2400
Pittsburgh, PA 15220
(412) 429-1151
FAX (412) 429-0211
BA,NT,Cosm. Surg.

David Goldstein, MD
9401 McKnight Rd., #301-B
Pittsburgh, PA 15237
(412) 366-6780
Email: DAVIDG25@aol.com
A,DD,MM,NT,PM,PMR

Edward C. Kondrot, MD,
BPCT
239 4th Avenue
Pittsburgh, PA 15222
(412) 281-0447
FAX (412) 281-3660
CT,NT,Homeopathy

QUAKERTOWN

Harold Buttram, MD, APCT
5724 – Clymer Road
Quakertown, PA 18951
(215) 536-1890
A,CT,FP,NT

William G. Kracht, DO, BPCT
5724 Clymer Rd.
Quakertown, PA 18951
(215) 536-1890
Email: bkracht@woodmed.com
A,CT,FP,NT,OS,YS

SCRANTON

Okhee Won, MD, BPCT
1822 Mulberry St.
Scranton, PA 18510
(570) 969-8165
FAX (570) 969-8729
Email: owon@clinical.com
Pathology

SPRINGFIELD

Walter W. Schwartz, DO
471 Baltimore Pike
Springield, PA 19064
(610) 604-4800
FAX (610) 604-4815
Email: smile7@op.net
CD,CT,IM

TOPTON

Conrad G. Maulfair, Jr., DO,
FACAM, APC
P.O. Box 98
403 North Main St.
Topton, PA 19562
(610) 682-2104
FAX (610) 682-9781
coleenmaulfair@enter.net
A,CT,HGL

WEST MIDDLESEX

Robert D. Multari, DO
15 Elliott Rd.
West Middlesex, PA 16159
(412) 981-2246
A,CD,DD,DIA,GE,IM

WILLIAMSPORT

Francis M. Powers, Jr., MD
1201 Grampian Blvd., #3-A
3rd Floor
Williamsport, PA 17701
(570) 322-6450
FAX (570) 322-0648
CT,NT,OME,YS, Therapeutic
Radiology

WYNCOTE

Steven C. Halbert, MD, APCT
1442 Ashbourne Rd.
Wyncote, PA 19095
(215) 886-7842
FAX (215) 887-1921
steven.halbert@mail.tju.edu
A,CT,IM,NT,YS

YARDLEY

Anca Bereanu, MD
401 Floral Vale Blvd.
Yardley, PA 19067
(215) 504-9636
FAX (215) 504-1094
Neurology, HOM

RHODE ISLAND

NEWPORT

Dariusz J. Nasiek, MD
17 Friendship Street
Newport, RI 02840
(401) 846-1230
AN,PM,CT

SOUTH CAROLINA

CHARLESTON

Art M. LaBruce, MD
9231A Medical Plaza Dr.
N. Charleston, SC 29406
(843) 572-1771
FAX (843) 572-8962
A,CT,NT,PM,RHI,S

COLUMBIA

Connie G. Ross, MD, BPCT
2228 Airport Road
Columbia, SC 29169
(803) 796-1702
CT,NT,PM

James M. Shortt, MD, BPCT
3981 Edmund Hwy., #A
W. Columbia, SC 29170
(803) 755-0114
FAX (803) 755-0116
jimmydoc@mindspring.com
CT,Neural Therapy, P/S, Anti-
Aging

MARION

H.V. Coleman, MD
P.O. Box 1070
Marion, SC 29571
NO REFERRALS

MYRTLE BEACH

Peter Busse, MD
306 79th Ave., North
Myrtle Beach, SC 29572
(843) 449-5200
FAX (843) 447-6471
FP

SPARTANBURG

James Shortt, MD, BPCT
2500 Winchester Pl., #107
Spartanburg, SC 29301
(864) 595-2552
FAX (864) 595-2554
jimmydoc@mindspring.com
CT,Neural Therapy, P/S, Anti-
Aging

SOUTH DAKOTA

CUSTER

Dennis R. Wicks, MD
1 Holiday Trail, HCR 83, Box 21
Custer, SD 57730-9703
(605) 673-2689
GP,S

SIOUX FALLS

Harold J. Fletcher, MD
4601 S. Techlink Circle
Sioux Falls, SD 57106
(605) 362-8256
FAX (605) 362-8293
CT,FP,GE,NT,P/S

WATERTOWN

Mary Goepfert, MD –
RETIRED
P.O. Box 513
Watertown, SD 57201
NO REFERRALS

TENNESSEE

ATHENS

H. Joseph Holliday, MD,
FACAM, APCT
1005 W. Madison Ave.
Athens, TN 37303
(423) 744-7540
FAX (423) 745-4898
CT,CD,CS,S

CHATTANOOGA

Charles C. Adams, MD, BPCT
3739 Hixson Pike
Chattanooga, TN 37415
(423) 875-0999
Email: drprevent@aol.com
IM,CT,NT,A,Anti-Aging Med.

Robert A. Burkich, MD, APCT
707 Signal Mountain Blvd.
Chattanooga, TN 37405
(423) 266-4474
FAX (423) 266-4464
Email: DrStayWell@aol.com
CT,GP,PM

HIXSON

Mark T. Simpson, MD
4513 Hixon Pike, #102
Hixson, TN 37343
(423) 877-7999
FAX (423) 877-7901
FP,CT,PM

JOHNSON CITY

David Livingston, MD, BPCT
108 West Springbrook Dr.
Johnson City, TN 37604
(423) 282-1888
FAX (423) 282-0921
BA,CD,CT,FP,PM

KINGSPORT

Pickens Gantt, MD
#307 – 2204 Pavilion Dr.
Kingsport, TN 37660
(423) 392-6330
FAX (423) 392-6053
CT,NT,PM,END,GYN

David Livingston, MD, BPCT
1567 N. Eastman Rd., #4
Kingsport, TN 37604
(423) 245-6671
FAX (423) 245-0966
BA,CD,CT,FP,PM

KNOXVILLE

William O. Murray, MD
7328 Middlebrook Pike
Knoxville, TN 37909
(865) 769-2600
FAX (865) 769-2616
FP

MEMPHIS

Jerry R. Floyd, MD
1027 Whitney Ave.
Memphis, TN 38127
(901) 353-5009
FAX (901) 353-6549
FP,GP,PM,CT

NASHVILLE

Robert A. Burkich, MD, APCT
388 Harding Place, Suite C
Nashville, TN 37211
(615) 445-7993
FAX (615) 445-7995
Email: edwin48@aol.com
CT,GP,PM

Stephen L. Reisman, MD
2325 Crestmoor Rd., #P-150
Nashville, TN 37215
(615) 298-2820
FAX (615) 298-2770
CT,GP,GHL,NT,PM,YS

OLD HICKORY

Russell Hunt, MD
1415 Robinson Road
Old Hickory, TN 37138
(615) 541-0400
FAX (615) 847-4142
Email: rjhunt@bellsouth.net
CT,FP,PM,NT,WR,A

TEXAS

AMARILLO

Gerald Parker, DO
4714 S. Western
Amarillo, TX 79109
(806) 355-8263
FAX (806) 355-8796
A,AC,AR,CT,GP,HO

John T. Taylor, DO
4714 S. Western
Amarillo, TX 79109
(806) 355-8263
FAX (806) 355-8796
A,AC,AR,CT,GP,HO

ARLINGTON

R. E. Liverman, DO
801 W. Road to Six Flags, #417
Arlington, TX 76012
(817) 461-7774
FAX (817) 801-5600
A,CT,NT,OSM,OME,DD,PO

AUSTIN

Ted Edwards Jr., MD
4201 Bee Caves Rd., #B-112
Austin, TX 78746
(512) 327-4886
GE,IM,PM, Sports Med., CT

Vladimir Rizov, MD, BPCT
911 W. Anderson Lane, #205
Austin, TX 78757
(512) 451-8149
FAX (512) 451-0895
AR,CT,DD,DIA,GP,IM

CONROE

Frank O. McGehee Jr., MD, BPCT
900 West Davis
Conroe, TX 77301
(936) 756-3366
drmcgehee@gateway.net
PM,NT

DALLAS

Chris J. Renna, DO
2706 Fairmount Street
Dallas, TX 75204
(214) 303-1888
END,FP,MM,NT,OS,PM

EULESS

Marina Johnson, MD
350 Westpark Way, #210
Euless, TX 76040
(817) 358-0663
FAX (817) 358-9163
END,PM,NT,IM,MM,YS

FORT WORTH

Barry L. Beaty, DO
4455 Camp Bowie, #211
Fort Worth, TX 76107
(817) 737-6464
FAX (817) 737-2858
CT,FP,PM,PMR

Gerald Harris, DO, BPCT
1002 Montgomery, #103
Fort Worth, TX 76107
(817) 732-2878
FAX (817) 732-9315
CT, Pain Mgmt.,P/S

Joseph F. McWherter, MD, BPCT
1307 – 8th Ave., #207
Fort Worth, TX 76104
(817) 926-2511
FAX (817) 924-0167
GYN,OBS,END,S,NT, Nat.
Hormones for W

Ricardo Tan, MD
3220 North Freeway, #106
Fort Worth, TX 76111
(817) 626-1933
AC,AU,CT,FP,NT,PM

GRAPEVINE

Constantine A. Kotsanis, MD
1600 W. College St., #260
Grapevine, TX 76051
(817) 481-6342
FAX (817) 488-8903
A,AC,CT,DD,NT,PM

HARLINGEN

Robert R. Somerville, MD
712 N. 77 Sunshine Strip, #21
Harlingen, TX 78550
(956) 428-0757
FAX (956) 428-8560
CT,HGL,NT,RHI,YS

HOUSTON

Robert Battle, MD, APCT
9910 Long Point
Houston, TX 77055
(713) 932-0552
FAX (713) 932-0551
A,BA,CD,CT,FP,HGL

Jerome L. Borochoff, MD
8830 Long Point, Suite 504
Houston, TX 77055
(713) 461-7517
FAX (713) 935-0040
CD,CT,FP,HO,PM

Jacqueline Brown, MD, PBCT
4504 Caroline Street
Houston, TX 77004
(713) 523-2334
FAX (713) 523-2602
GYN,CT,NT,OBS,PM,YS

Moe Kakvan, MD, APCT
3838 Hillcroft, #415
Houston, TX 77057
(713) 780-7019
FAX (713) 780-9783
CT,PM

Ji-Zhou (Joseph) Kang, MD (H)
6103 Corporate Drive
Houston, TX 77036
(702) 798-2992
A,AC,GP,IM,NT

HOUSTON

Steven J. Levy, DO, BPCT
1140 Westmont, #300
Houston, TX 77015
(713) 451-4100
FAX (713) 451-0010
DD,GER,HGL,IM,NT, OS

Gilbert Manso, MD
5177 Richmond Ave., #215
Houston, TX 77056
(713) 840-9355
FAX (713) 840-9468
CT,DD,GP,HGL,MM,YS

Marina M. Pearsall, MD, PhD
1213 Hermann Dr., #545
Houston, TX 77004
(713) 522-4037
FAX (713) 522-4872
CD,CT,DIA,IM,PMR, Weight Reduction

R.G. Tannerya, MD
9627 Pagewood Lane
Houston, TX 77063
NO REFERRALS

Stephen Joel Weiss, MD
7333 North Freeway, #100
Houston, TX 77076
(713) 691-0737
FAX (713) 695-0105
Ortho Surg

HUNTSVILLE

Frank O. McGehee Jr., MD, BPCT
1901 — 22nd Street
Huntsville, TX 77340
(936) 291-3351
FAX (936) 291-3519
PM,NT

IRVING

Frances J. Rose, MD
1701 W. Walnut Hill, #200
Irving, TX 75038
(972) 594-1111
FAX (972) 518-1867
A,AC,CT,FP,HGL,NT,PD,PM

JEFFERSON

Donald Ray Whitaker, DO
210 E. Elizabeth St.
Jefferson, TX 75657
(903) 665-7781
FAX (903) 665-7887
drwhitaker@drwhitakersvitamins.com
PM,NT,CT,WR,YS

KIRBYVILLE

John L. Sessions, DO, APCT
1609 South Margaret
Kirbyville, TX 75956
(409) 423-2166
CT,IM,OSM

LONGVIEW

Patricia F. Sanders, MD
472 East Loop 281, Suite B
Longview, TX 75605
(903) 236-0033
FAX (903) 234-1437
A,CT,GYN,NT,RHU

MCALLEN

Michael R. Kilgore, MD, BPCT
3600 N. 23rd. #201
McAllen, TX 78501
(210) 687-6196
CT,FP,GP,IM,PMR

PASADENA

Robert Baylis II, DO
5912 Spencer Hwy.
Pasadena, TX 77505
(713) 926-6229
FAX (713) 926-9292
FP,PM,OS,NT,YS

PLEASANTON

Gerald Phillips, MD
218 W. Goodwin Street
Pleasanton, TX 78064
(210) 569-2118
FAX (210) 569-5958
CD,CT,FP,HGL,NT,PM

ROWLETT

Robert J. Gilbard, MD
3809 Main Street
Rowlett, TX 75088
(972) 463-1744
FAX (972) 463-8243
GYN,CT,NT

SAN ANGELO

Benjamin Thurman, MD
610 S. Abe Street, #A
San Angelo, TX 76903
(915) 481-0596
FAX (915) 481-0597
AC,HOM,NT,Neuro Sclerotherapy

SAN ANTONIO

Daniel J. Boyle II, DO, BPCT
11118 Wurzbach, #204
San Antonio, TX 78230
(210) 690-6393
FAX (210) 690-6394
GP,OS,PMR,P/S,Emerg.Med.

Linda L. Welch, DO
11312 Perrin Beitel
San Antonio, TX 78217
(210) 946-5633
FAX (210) 946-5632
CT,FP,PM,P/S

SEABROOK

Ronald M. Davis, MD, BPCT,
RETIRED
5002 Todville
Seabrook, TX 77586
NO REFERRALS

VICTORIA

Rolando G. Arafiles Jr., MD,
BPCT
202 James Coleman Dr., #4
Victoria, TX 77904
(361) 570-3641
FAX (361) 570-3644
A,DIA,FP,NT,GER,PM

WACO

William P. Coleman, MD
504 Meadow Lake Ctr.
Waco, TX 76712
(254) 776-7444
FAX (254) 776-9729
CT,GP,NT,PM

WICHITA FALLS

Thomas Roger Humphrey, MD
2400 Rushing
Wichita Falls, TX 76308
(940) 766-4329
FAX (940) 767-3227
BA,FP,GP,HYP

ZAPATA

Ernest Cabrera, MD
P.O. Box 68
Zapata, TX 78076
NO REFERRALS

UTAH

ALPINE

Dianne Farley-Jones, MD
70 E. Red Pine Drive
Alpine, UT 84004
(801) 756-9444
FAX (801) 763-1070
FP

DRAPER

Dennis Harper, DO, BPCT
12226 S. 1000 East, #10
Draper, UT 84020
(801) 277-5000
FAX (801) 277-5200
A,CT,OSM,YS

PROVO

Dennis Remington, MD
1675 N. Freedom Blvd., Suite
11E
Provo, UT 84604
(801) 373-8500
FAX (801) 373-3426
A,CT,FP,Env. Med.

ST. GEORGE

Dennis Harper, DO, BPCT
321 North Mall Dr., L-103
St. George, UT 84790
(435) 674-3500
FAX (435) 673-7740
A,CT,OSM,YS

VERMONT

Essex Junction

Charles Anderson, MD
175 Peart Street
Essex Junction, VT 05452
A,FP,NT,YS

VIRGINIA

ALDIE

Norman W. Levin, MD, APCT
39070 John Mosby Hwy.
P.O. Box 107
Aldie, VA 20105-0107
(703) 327-2434
FAX (703) 327-2729
CT,IM,PM,RHU

ALEXANDRIA

Manjit R. Bajwa, MD
6391 Little River Turnpike
Alexandria, VA 22312
(703) 941-3606
FAX (703) 658-6415
CT,DD,END,GP,HO, MM

ARLINGTON

Andrew Baer, MD
2300 S. 24th Road, #242
Arlington, VA 22206
(703) 979-5035
FAX (208) 475-7629
IM

CHESAPEAKE

Ernest Aubrey Murden Jr.,
MD, BPCT
4020 Raintree Rd., #C
Chesapeake, VA 23321
(757) 488-2080
FAX (757) 405-3025
A,CT,NT,RHI

FALLS CHURCH

Aldo M. Rosemblat, MD, APCT
6316 Castle Place, #200
Falls Church, VA 22044
(703) 241-8989
FAX (703) 532-6247
AC,S

HINTON

Harold Huffman, MD, APCT
P.O. Box 197
Hinton, VA 22831
(540) 867-5154
CT,FP,PM

LOUISA

David G. Schwartz, MD
P.O. Box 532
Louisa, VA 23093
(540) 967-2050
CT,FP,NT

NELLYSFORD

Mitchell A. Fleisher, MD
P.O. Box 303
Rockfish Ctr., Suite One, SR 664
Nellysford, VA 22958
(804) 361-1896
FAX (804) 361-1928
CT,FP,MM,NT,PM, HOM

RICHMOND

Peter C. Gent, DO, APCT
2621 Promenade Pkwy.
Midlothian, VA 23113
(804) 897-8566
FAX (804) 897-8569
CT,GP,OSM

Mary N. Megson, MD
7229 Forest Ave., #211
Richmond, VA 23226
(804) 673-9128
FAX (804) 673-9195
Autism,ADHD,Learning
Disability

ROANOKE

Joan M. Resk, DO
5249 Clearbrook Lane
Roanoke, VA 24014
(540) 776-8331
FAX (540) 776-8303
CD,CT,DD,OSM,NT,PM

TROUT DALE

Eduardo Castro, MD
799 Ripshin Road, P.O. Box 44
Trout Dale, VA 24378
(540) 677-3631
FAX (540) 677-3843
Email: mrc@drcranton.com
A,CD,CT,HO,NT,PM

Elmer M. Cranton, MD,
FACAM, APCT
799 Ripshin Road, Box 44
Trout Dale, VA 24378
(540) 677-3631
FAX (540) 677-3843
drcranton@drcranton.com
A,CD,CT,FP,HO,NT

VIRGINIA BEACH

Robert A. Nash, MD, FACAM, APCT
5589 Greenwich Rd., #175
Virginia Beach, VA 23462
(757) 490-9311
FAX (757) 490-9266
AC,CT,NT,PM,Neuro.,Pain Med.

WARRENTON

James B. Hutt Jr., MD
550 Broadview Ave., Rm. 202
Warrenton, VA 20186
(540) 347-0474
CT,GP,OPH

YORKTOWN

Robert McLean
111 Lord North Court
Yorktown, VA 23693

WASHINGTON

BELLEVUE

David Buscher, MD
1603 – 116th N.E., Suite 112
Bellevue, WA 98004-3825
(425) 453-0288
FAX (425) 455-0076
Env. Med./Cin. Ecol,GP,NT

Betty Sy Go, MD, APCT
15611 Bel-Red Road
Bellevue, WA 98105
(425) 881-2224
FAX (425) 881-2216
Email: bpsygo@pol.net
A,AC,CT,FP,NT,PM

BELLINGHAM

Andrew Pauli, MD
116 Key Street
Bellingham, WA 98225
(360) 671-1369
FAX (360) 671-0981
DD,END,NT,PM,PO,P

ELK

Stanley B. Covert, MD, BPCT
42207 N. Sylvan Road
Elk, WA 99009
(509) 292-2748
CT,FP,GP,Emerg.

FEDERAL WAY

Thomas A. Dorman, MD, APCT
2505 South 320th St., #100
Federal Way, WA 98003
(253) 529-9781
FAX (253) 529-9782
Email: tdorman@nwlink.com
CD,CT,IM,P/S

George Koss, DO
1014 South 320th Street
Federal Way, WA 98003
(253) 839-4100
FAX (253) 941-6116
georgekoss@hotmail.com
FP,PM,NT,HGL,CD,CT

KENT

Jonathan Wright, MD
515 West Harrison, #200
Kent, WA 98032
(253) 854-4900
FAX (253) 850-5639
A,CT,FP,MM,NT,END

KIRKLAND

Jonathan Collin, MD, FACAM, APCT
12911 120th Ave. N.E., #A-50,
POB 8099
Kirkland, WA 98034
(425) 820-0547
FAX (425) 820-0259
CT,NT,PM

PORT TOWNSEND

Jonathan Collin, MD, FACAM, APCT
911 Tyler Street
Port Townsend, WA 98368
(360) 385-4555
FAX (360) 385-0699
CT,NT,PM

J. Douwe Rienstra, MD BPCT
242 Monroe Street
Port Townsend, WA 98368
(360) 385-5688
FAX (360) 385-5142
Email: Medical@olympus.net
GP,MM,NT,PM

RICHLAND

Geoffrey S. Ames, MD
750 Swift Blvd., #1
Richland, WA 99397
(509) 943-3934
CT,MM,NT,Env. Med.,HOM,
Dermatology

SEATTLE

Ralph Golan, MD
7522 – 20th Ave., N.E.
Seattle, WA 98115
(206) 524-8966
FAX (206) 524-8951
CT,CD,END,GE,NT,YS

SPOKANE

William Corell, MD
3424 Grand Blvd., South
Spokane, WA 99203
(509) 838-5800
FAX (509) 838-4042
CT,FP,NT,PM,HGL,YS,MM

Burton B. Hart, DO
E. 12104 Main
Spokane, WA 99206
(509) 927-9922
FAX (509) 926-2011
CT,PM,OSM,P/S

VANCOUVER

Steve Kennedy, MD, BPCT
615 S.E. Chkalov, #14
Vancouver, WA 98683
(360) 256-4566
FAX (360) 253-3060
Reconstructive Surgery
(hand),CT,PM

YELM

Elmer M. Cranton, MD,
FACAM, APCT
503 First Street So., #1
P.O. Box 5100
Yelm, WA 98597-5100
(360) 458-1061
FAX (360) 458-1661
drcranton@drcranton.com
A,CD,CT,FP,HO,NT

Stephen Olmstead, MD
503 First St. South, #1
Yelm, WA 98597
(360) 458-1061
FAX (360) 458-1661
Email: aesclepios@att.net
CD,IM

WEST VIRGINIA

BECKLEY

Prudencio Corro, MD, BPCT
251 Stanaford Rd.
Beckley, WV 25801
(304) 252-0775
A,CT,RHI

CHARLESTON

Steve M. Zekan, MD
1208 Kanawha Blvd. E.
Charleston, WV 25301
(304) 343-7559
FAX (304) 343-1219
CT,NT,PM,S

HURRICANE

John P. MacCallum, MD
3855 Teays Valley Road
Hurricane, WV 25526
(304) 757-3368
FAX (304) 757-2402
CT,MM,P,PM

Dallas B. Bartin, DO, BPCT
1401 Hospital Dr., #302
Hurricane, WV 25526
(304) 757-8090
FAX (304) 757-8079
FP,OS

SUMMERSVILLE

John R. Ray, DO
3029 Webster Rd.
Summersville, WV 26651
(304) 872-6583
FP

WISCONSIN

DELAFIELD

Carol Uebelacker, MD
700 Milwaukee St.
Delafield, WI 53018
(262) 646-4600
FAX (262) 646-4215
A,CD,BA,CT,FP,GYN

GREEN BAY

Eleazar M. Kadile, MD, APCT
1538 Bellevue St.
Green Bay, WI 54311
(920) 468-9442
FAX (920) 468-9714
A,CT,P

LA CROSSE

Patrick J. Scott, MD
3454 Losey Blvd. S.
La Crosse, WI 54601
(608) 785-0038
FAX (608) 782-5959
A,CT,GP,NT,PM,YS

MILWAUKEE

J. Allan Robertson, Jr., DO,
APCT
1011 N. Mayfair Rd., #301
Milwaukee, WI 53226
(414) 302-1011
FAX (414) 302-1010
CT,FP,GP,NT,OS,YS

Carol Uebelacker, MD
5404-A North Lovers Lane Rd.
Milwaukee, WI 53225
(414) 466-2002
FAX (414) 466-2855
A,CD,BA,CT,FP,GYN

Jerry N. Yee, DO
2505 N. Mayfair Rd., #104
Milwaukee, WI 53226
(414) 258-6282
BA,CT,GP,OSM

WISCONSIN DELLS

Robert S. Waters, MD, APCT
Race & Vine Streets, Box 357
Wisconsin Dells, WI 53965
(608) 254-7178
FAX (608) 253-7139
Email: rwaters@mwt.net
CT,PM,OME

WYOMING

Gillette

Rebecca Painter, MD, APCT
201 West Lakeway, #300
Gillette, WY 82718
(307) 682-0330
FAX (307) 686-8118
Email: rapmd@vcn.com
CD,CT,DIA,IM,PUD,RHU

APPENDIX B

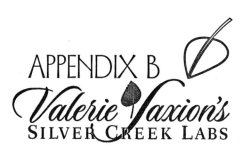

Valerie Saxion's
SILVER CREEK LABS

AQUA FLORA

A state-of-the-art, high-potency homeopathic that successfully fights *Candida Albicans* in record time. Employs the same principle as all effective vaccines.

BODY OXYGEN

A pleasant-tasting nutritional supplement that is meticulously manufactured with cold pressed aloe vera. The aloe is used as a stabilized carrier for numerous nutritional constituents, including magnesium peroxide and pure anaerocidal oxygen, hawthorne berry, ginkgo biloba, ginseng, and St. John's Wort. It helps to naturally fight infections, inflammation, and degeneration by taking oxygen in at the cellular level. It also commonly helps in colon cleansing, regular elimination, and provides a feeling of increased energy and mental alertness.

BOVINE THYROID

A naturally safe way to boost your natural production of thyroxin without the risk of various side effects. The thyroid is responsible for everything from your metabolism to your sex drive. If you suspect you are among the one out of every four Americans who suffer from an under-active thyroid, consult your physician and consider this as a natural alternative.

CALCIUM/MAGNESIUM

The USDA reports that 78 percent of adult women and 56 percent of adult men don't get enough calcium from their diets. The majority of teenagers are also lacking this vital nutrient. Our liquid Calcium/Magnesium is pleasant tasting and supplies the proper ratio designed for optimal absorption, essential for the support of healthy bones and teeth.

CANDICID FORTE

This product, with its powerful agents that contain liver and gastrointestinal herbs to maximize its performance, has been greatly improved by using more consistent extracts and the addition of both berberine sulfate and oregano extract.

CHINESE HERB STIMULATING SHAMPOO BY PETER LAMAS

All-natural and botanically rich stimulating shampoo empowered by 50 Chinese herbs. Gently removes hair follicle-blockage and debris that can slow growth and eventually cause premature hair loss. Helps alleviate dryness, flakes, and itching!

COLLOIDAL SILVER

A universal germ killer and natural antibiotic. It has proven superior to every other silver because of its ultra-fine particle size in a cubical shape, positively charged with 30 to 35 parts per million. It contains no salt, electrolytes, or binders with zero contamination. A partial list of bacteria/viruses tested and neutralized with Colloidal Silver in the laboratory were Lyme, Herpes, Legionnaire, Staphylococcus, Aureus, Salmonella, Choleraesuis, Streptococci, Warts, Pseudomonas, Aeruginosa,

Neisseria Gonorrhea, Gardnerella Vaginalis, Gangrene, and Candida. Great for burns as well.

COLLOIDAL SILVER NASAL SPRAY

Most users describe this nasal spray as miraculous and life-changing and extraordinarily effective! No nasal burning, attacks infection, reduces swelling, and aids in fast healing.

COLLOIDAL MINERALS

These minerals are a concentrated liquid extracted from a very rare, ancient deposit of plant origin. Our special low-temperature processing makes these minerals available in a colloidal state with pure water. No synthetics, coloring, or preservatives are added. Mined from the richest source in the United States for over 70 years. We guarantee over 70 colloidal minerals in each serving.

COLON CLEANSE

Super herbal cleanse for those times when your eliminative system is not what it should be. Also excellent to assist in detoxifying and cleansing your body.

CLUSTERED WATER

Dr. Lorenzen's Clustered Water is probably the greatest breakthrough in health science product development in this century. Clustered Water, produced at home using one ounce of solution to one gallon of steam-distilled water, replenishes the most vital support for all cellular DNA and the 4,000 plus enzymes that are involved in every metabolic process in your body. Increases nutrient absorption by up to 600 percent, which means your vitamins and organic foods will deliver far more vital nutrients to your body. Replicates the powerful healing waters of the earth! Excellent for cleaning out lymphatic fluids! Comes in a C-400 formula for those who are generally healthy and detoxed, and a SBX formula for the immune-compromised.

CREATION'S BOUNTY

Simply the best, pleasant-tasting, green, whole, raw, organic food supplement available—a blend of whole, raw, organic herbs and grains, principally amaranth, brown rice, spirulina, and flaxseed. This combination of live foods with live enzymes assists your body in the digestion of foods void of enzymes. You will gain vital nutrients, protein, carbohydrates, and good fats to nourish your body and brain, resulting in extra energy and an immunity boost as well. It is a whole food, setting it apart from other green foods on the market.

DIGESTIVE ENZYMES

Digestion is the means by which food is broken down in order for the body to utilize it. If this process is inhibited for any reason, it may be necessary to take a supplement to ensure sufficient digestion. Bloating, belching, burning, or flatulence immediately after meals are common symptoms of low gastric acidity. So are indigestion, diarrhea, constipation, multiply food allergies, and nausea after taking supplements. Research has shown that the ingredients in our Digestive Enzymes have proven to be very effective in the first stages of (stomach) digestion.

ESSENTIAL FATTY ACIDS

Without the "good fats" in our diet, our brain as well as our body suffers multiple consequences. ADD, ADHD, and Alzheimer patients, for instance, all lack the essential fatty acids. However, you can reverse this deficit simply by adding the Essential Fatty Acids to your diet and benefit by increasing the "good fats" in your daily regimen.

FAT MAGNET

This revolutionary formula includes LipoSan Ultra brand Chitosan, which has three times more fat-absorbing activity than other Chitosan products. Fat Magnet possesses a positive charge that actually attracts negatively charged fat. This electrostatic process helps remove unwanted fat from the foods you eat and gently eliminates it from your system. Can be taken with meals, offering a convenient and effective way to meet your weight-loss goals.

GREAT LEGS

Millions of Americans, mostly women, suffer with varicose or spider veins, leg swelling, and discomfort due to poor circulation caused by venous insufficiency. For years the French have used the Great Legs formula to increase blood flow to the legs and feet and to reduce the prominence of leg veins. All natural Great Legs contains a special plant extract, Ruscus aculeatus, that causes the smooth fibers of the veins to contract, allowing oxygenated, nutrient-rich blood to flow more freely to the lower extremities. With regular use, it can improve the look of your skin, reduce the prominence of varicose veins, curtail swelling, cramps, and tingling, and actually invigorate lower extremities so legs feel lighter and more energized.

HAPPY CAMPER

The original "feel good" formula that was one of the first all-natural herbal mood products to include Kava Kava and Passion Flower in a special blend that helps you relax and reduces anxiety. This sophisticated blend of select herbs will lift your spirit and improve your attitude and, unlike single-ingredient mood products, provides you with a true sense of well-being.

HYDROGEN PEROXIDE

Non-hazardous, food-grade, liquid oxygen used for a variety of purposes, including the famous "Oxygen Bath." Ask for our free booklet on H_2O_2.

HYDROGEN PEROXIDE GEL

Bad bacteria (anaerobic) can't live in the presence of oxygen, which is why hospitals around the world use hydrogen peroxide to clean and sterilize wounds in the prevention of infections. Our gel goes one step further by binding the peroxide to the area of treatment with pure glycerin, allowing the active ingredient the extra time it needs to work.

MENOPAUSE RELIEF CREAM

This is a natural progesterone/phytoestrogen cream. Unlike synthetic estrogen, phytoestrogens do not increase the risk of breast cancer. If you are between the ages of 40 and 55 and have symptoms of regular or irregular menses, irritability, anxiety, depression, mood swings, breast tenderness two weeks before menses, hot flashes, night sweats, insomnia, vaginal dryness, headaches, fuzzy thinking, short-term memory loss, frequent urinary tract infections, dry hair or hair loss, or low sex drive, this product is for you.

NIACIN B-3

So needed, so overlooked, so simple, and so inexpensive! Great for circulation, skin, heart, blood flow, and high cholesterol. The National Cholesterol Foundation ranks Niacin over name-brand pharmaceutical cholesterol drugs.

OLIVE LEAF EXTRACT

For centuries the olive leaf has been used in traditional medicine as an antiseptic, anti-hypertensive, astringent, fever reducer, and for numerous other purposes. In 1962 an Italian researcher reported that oleuropein, a bitter glycoside found abundantly in olive leaf, was able to lower blood pressure in mammals. This sparked further research, which proved olive leaf to be a potent anti-microbial as well as antibacterial and anti-viral. This investigation included viruses such as herpes, vaccinia, pseudorabies, Newcastle, Cossacloe A21, Monloney sarcoma, leukemia, influenza, and many more.

ORGANIC BODY POLISH

Sea salt has been known for centuries to detoxify, heal, and restore the body to balance. Our Organic Body Polish is loaded with sea salt and organic herbs, which acts like a magnet, pulling heavy metals and low radiation from the body, while leaving you feeling like silk. Comes in Calming, Warming, and Clearing.

ORTHOBIOTIC

A specially formulated intestinal bacteria supplement that promotes optimal health and nutrient absorption by reestablishing the ideal gut micro-flora. Ingredients include non-pathogenic cultered organisms from the families Bacillus, Arthrobacter, Azotobacter, Pseudomnas, Chaetomium, Streptomyces, Trichoderma, Berticillium, and Aspergillus.

OXYGEN SUBLINGUAL SPRAY

A concentrated form of Body Oxygen™ that quickly delivers oxygen through the thin lining under your tongue. It is packaged as a convenient, easy-to-carry spray, delivering a powerful dose of oxygen that stimulates mental activity and invigorates your body while delivering numerous herbal benefits when you are "on the go."

PH STICKS

Knowing your PH level is imperative. Disease thrives in an acidic environment. By checking your PH on a regular basis, you can make the adjustments needed to bring your body up to a more alkaline state.

PROHELP

A natural progesterone cream. If you are between the ages of 14 and 40 and have symptoms of irritability, anxiety, depression, mood swings, food cravings, breast tenderness two weeks before menses, and menstrual cramps, this product is for you.

RADIANT-C FACE & BODY WASH
BY PETER LAMAS

Packed with a highly potent 7 percent L-Ascorbic Vitamin C, Radiant C is designed to brighten, clarify, and retexturize aging skin. It delivers energy without irritating or dehydrating, gently loosens and removes makeup, dead skin cells, oils, and gives a mild lather that leaves you looking and feeling fresher from head to toe. Best of all, there are no harmful chemicals.

REACTED SELENIUM

Selenium is a very important trace element that also functions as a powerful antioxidant. Recent research has shown that appropriate selenium intake is associated with optimum health.

RICE PROTEIN VOLUMIZING SHAMPOO
BY PETER LAMAS

Rice protein strengthens and expands the diameter of the hair shaft to create thicker, more luxurious hair.

SMART-PILL

The IQ-Maximizer, 100 percent natural and herbal. The student's best help for mental clarity, concentration, creativity, and optimum brain power. May restore normal brain function for attention deficit disorder, Alzheimer's, Parkinson's, and other neurological concerns. May reduce cortisol levels, which is one of the main causes of depression and a key to muscle building. May eliminate constipation and promote regular toxin excretion.

SOY BALANCING CONDITIONER
BY PETER LAMAS

Soy-rich conditioner detangles and protects hair of every type, even hair that has been chemically treated.

SOY HYDRATING SHAMPOO
BY PETER LAMAS

Nature's protein revitalizing shampoo designed to restore and strengthen chemically treated, dry, weak, or damaged hair.

SUPER FLEX BACK FORMULA

Reduces pain and inflammation! Contains Turmeric, ginger, and Protykin trans-reversatrol imperative for phytonutrients that inhibit the COX-2 enzyme. Also included in this unique blend is Boswellin, which is known to reduce inflammation, and Kava Kava and magnesium to relax back muscles and break the pain cycle. In addition, it contains MSM and Glucosamine to repair damaged connective tissue. The combination in Super Flex makes this product complete for back support and pain!

ULTRA DIET PEP

Maximum strength formula contains some of the most powerful thermogenic herbs in the world, tempered with a sophisticated blend of ingredients that balance the energizing effect. In addition, it offers special nutrients for dieters, including Dyna Chrome Chromium to promote proper blood sugar metabolism so you don't crave between-meal snacks. Also contains the popular "dieters vitamins," B-6 and B-12, as well as Pantothenic Acid to help manage the stress of dieting.

VEGGIE WASH

A safe, easy, and effective way to clean your produce and reduce your risk of chemical toxicity and parasites. Unfortunately, our foods are sprayed with so many things to keep them fresh and get them to market, we have no idea what all may really be on them.

WHEAT GRASS DEEP CLEANSING SHAMPOO BY PETER LAMAS

A naturally effective, gentle cleanser that removes residue and debris without stripping out the moisture and vitality while keeping hair color looking vibrant. Gentle enough to use every day.

YOUR DAILY MULTI VITAMIN & MINERAL

An all-natural, food-based vitamin and mineral supplement without iron and copper. Contains the nutrients you need to survive in a toxic world that has been depleted by harmful chemical spraying and failure to rotate crops.

To contact Silver Creek Laboratories for a complete catalog and order form, call (817) 236-8557, or fax (817) 236-5411, or write us at 7000 Lake Country Dr., Fort Worth, TX 76179.